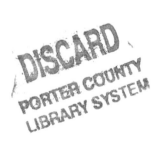

THE MYTHS OF MODERN MEDICINE

THE MYTHS OF MODERN MEDICINE

The Alarming Truth about American Health Care

John Leifer

ROWMAN & LITTLEFIELD
Lanham • Boulder • New York • London

Published by Rowman & Littlefield
A wholly owned subsidary of The Rowman & Littlefield Publishing Group, Inc.
4501 Forbes Boulevard, Suite 200, Lanham, Maryland 20706
www.rowman.com

16 Carlisle Street, London W1D 3BT, United Kingdom

British Library Cataloguing in Publication Information Available

Library of Congress Cataloging-in-Publication Data

Leifer, John, 1957– author.
The myths of modern medicine : the alarming truth about American health care / John Leifer.
p. ; cm.
Alarming truth about American health care
Includes bibliographical references and index.
Summary: The American healthcare system is terminally ill, astonishingly expensive, remarkably variable in quality and incapable of stemming the rising tide of chronic illnesses in our population. This book strips away the elaborately constructed myths that conceal the ugly underbelly of healthcare and lays bare the truth about an industry that serves special interest groups far better than it serves its patients. Just as the Affordable Care Act begins to change the healthcare landscape, Leifer offers a survival guide for anyone entering the healthcare system.
ISBN 978-1-4422-2595-4 (cloth : alk. paper)—ISBN 978-1-4422-2596-1 (electronic)
I. Title. II. Title: Alarming truth about American health care.
[DNLM: 1. Delivery of Health Care—United States. 2. Quality of Health Care—United States. W 84 AA1]
RA412.2
368.38'200973—dc23
2014019040

CONTENTS

INTRODUCTION: THE END OF BLIND FAITH AND THE BEGINNING OF TRANSFORMATIONAL CHANGE IN HEALTH CARE

The American health care system is terminally ill. It is astonishingly expensive, remarkably variable in quality, and incapable of stemming the rising tide of chronic illness in our population.

Yet the majority of Americans believe it is the best system in the world and cling to the belief that, far from ailing, it delivers care superior to those of countries across the globe.

The system has obliged us by providing an elaborate set of myths about American health care that significantly shape our beliefs. These myths keep us blissfully ignorant about the true quality, safety, and value of the care we receive. This ignorance has a price: it leads us to draw erroneous conclusions about our conditions, fail to properly evaluate potential treatment options, and rarely question our providers' competency.

This book is based on the premise that consumer empowerment begins with an understanding of the true state of the health care system. Such knowledge increases not only the consumer's ability to receive appropriate care but also to take effective action to change the system. Armed with the correct information, consumers can make smart decisions for their health and the health of their families, as well as coalesce into social-action groups.

The book identifies ten myths that must be debunked to achieve a true appreciation for the condition of our system. It combines hard data with personal anecdotes collected over three decades of immersion in the industry. The identifying details for these anecdotes have been changed to maintain the anonymity of the individuals and institutions involved. In some cases, composite characters have been created.

The book also provides, where appropriate, specific steps that every consumer can take to optimize the quality, value, and effectiveness of the care they and their family receive. The epilogue serves as a consumer's guide to social action—for those readers wishing to play an active role in changing the dysfunctional health care system.

Throughout the book, the reader is reminded of their stewardship responsibility for their own health. Perhaps the most important lesson to be gleaned is the degree to which we can avoid encounters with the health care system by judiciously making smart decisions about our health.

If we are to heal the American health care system, we must understand how our false beliefs impair our ability to get efficient, effective, and safe care. Only then can we exercise stewardship responsibility for our own health. If patients understand how these myths influence their care, they might make better choices about their care, get more value from the system, and enjoy improved health and well-being. And if we all use the system differently, the process of reshaping it would begin to happen more naturally. We, as patients, can drive the reform of the system.

The Affordable Care Act has made health care reform one of the most hotly contested topics in America, but it does not address the core problems in our system. Meaningful health care reform isn't likely to happen as a result of legislative edicts from Washington. There is simply too much avarice and greed vying for its bounty. Reform will only happen when you as a patient, fully empowered with information, begin to assert your rights.

MYTH I
"THE UNITED STATES BOASTS THE BEST HEALTH CARE IN THE WORLD"

Betsy Lehman trusted her life to the American health care system. An award-winning journalist, Lehman was a rising star at the Boston Globe, *where she wrote extensively about health care issues. So when the mother of two was diagnosed with a particularly aggressive type of breast cancer, she knew instinctively where to go to receive outstanding care. Lehman selected a top-notch teaching hospital that has long been recognized as one of the nation's leading cancer hospitals.*

Lehman had done her research. She knew that her best chance for survival was to undergo an experimental stem-cell transplant designed to kill the cancer cells that were systemically circulating throughout her body. She also knew that cyclophosphamide, one of the chemotherapeutic agents she would be given before the transplant, would have a powerful effect on her body.

Lehman's treatment with cyclophosphamide would occur over a four-day period. Each day she would receive a precise dose that was determined by measuring the surface area of her body. In total, she was to receive slightly more than 6,500 milligrams of cyclophosphamide. Due to a cascade of errors, she received the full 6,500 milligram dose every day for four consecutive days.[1]

Despite the grievous error, Lehman appeared to be surviving the treatment—that is, until immediately before her scheduled discharge. Although she protested that something was desperately wrong, her care-

givers ignored her pleas for help. She never returned home. She died in the hospital from the massive overdose of the drugs purportedly used to heal her. There was no question as to culpability. The leadership of the hospital immediately accepted that responsibility.[2]

Ironically, according to an article in the New York Times, *an autopsy performed at the time of death showed no signs of cancer.*[3]

Betsy Lehman was a well-educated, well-known professional who sought care at a hospital considered to be one of the finest in the world. Yet she didn't survive her encounter. Is this American health care at its best?

Before concluding that such tragic outcomes are the rare outliers in health care, consider what *Time* magazine had to say shortly after Lehman's death: "Lehman's case," *Time* said, "is just one of a spate of medical foul-ups that have made headlines in recent weeks. In two Florida incidents, a doctor amputated the wrong foot of a diabetic man, and a hospital worker mistakenly turned off a stroke victim's breathing machine. In Michigan a surgeon doing a mastectomy removed a woman's healthy breast instead of the diseased one."[4]

Lehman's faith was misplaced twenty years ago, and our faith is arguably still misplaced today.

THE STRENGTH OF OUR CONVICTION

Faith is irrational. It transcends evidence and logic, and ultimately it requires the faithful to make a proverbial leap and accept anecdotal evidence in support of their convictions. Among the religiously devout, faith is an essential virtue, but faith can be misplaced.

Nowhere is this truer than in health care. Americans fervently cling to the belief that we have the best health care in the world, despite overwhelming evidence to the contrary.

The strength of these convictions was measured in a research study funded by the Robert Wood Johnson Foundation. The study's authors concluded that "there seems to be a routine genuflection to the widespread belief of U.S. quality excellence, even among experts."[5] The authors went on to note that, even in light of evidence regarding aberrantly high costs, the lack of adequate insurance coverage, and other issues, physicians and patients were unwavering in their faith.[6]

Why do we suspend critical thinking when it comes to health care? Because our beliefs comfort us—they reduce our sense of vulnerability to the inevitable onslaught of illness and injury that is part of the human condition. But our beliefs delude us. Our unquestioning faith is, in reality, a careless and reckless act that jeopardizes our well-being.

As we will discover together, our physicians are incredibly mortal and our health system fundamentally flawed. It is not a system that justifies our suspension of logic and abdication of personal responsibility for our health but, rather, one that demands our intense scrutiny.

The family of Betsy Lehman learned this lesson in the most painful way possible—at the cost of their loved one's life. Lehman sought treatment at one of the most prestigious facilities in America yet nonetheless experienced an unconscionable medical error that proved fatal. If it can happen in the corridors of our best medical institutions to well-known, public figures, it can happen to you.

Hospital-induced deaths represent the extreme end of the spectrum. There are far more insidious ways that our health care system fails us with regularity. The degree to which we are affected by this failure is somewhat a function of our discernment. Blind faith in our health care providers may have been the rule of order for our parents' generation, but it should not be for ours.

It is time to open our eyes and take an objective look at the "best" health care system in the world. But be forewarned: stripping away the false illusions that provide an unwarranted sense of security is painful.

U.S. HEALTH CARE VERSUS THE WORLD

A virtual army of researchers, working across multiple decades, have amassed a rich collection of data regarding how American health care compares to care delivered throughout the world. Their findings have appeared in innumerable peer-reviewed journals, books, magazines, and websites. Though the venues of publication have varied, the results have been amazingly consistent.

Almost categorically, experts agree on several major points: "The United States has nowhere near 'the best health care system in the world,' and that performance often falls markedly short of that of other countries"[7] ; and we pay dearly for what is arguably inferior care.[8]

Despite our narcissistic insistence that we are the world's top provider of care, we're actually many rungs down the ladder. The research study *Mirror, Mirror on the Wall* ranked U.S. health care dead last among seven industrialized nations—a finding repeated in studies conducted in 2004, 2006, 2007, and 2010. The nations included in these studies employed highly diverse systems and included Germany, the Netherlands, Australia, Canada, the United Kingdom, the United States, and New Zealand.[9] While we are quick to disparage other nations' systems, labeling them "socialized medicine" or other pejorative terms, our free-enterprise system is yielding an inferior product at a far greater cost.

Where's the proof of our inferiority? It exists in bucket loads . . . beginning with an examination of our relative life expectancy.

LIFE EXPECTANCY: AN EARLY INDICATOR OF HEALTH CARE QUALITY

We enter the world with a lease on life; for some, it is shorter than others. Poor hygiene, avoidable injuries, malnutrition, and the absence of appropriate care can have a marked impact on our time spent on Earth. One would assume, however, that in a wealthy nation with the most expensive health care system in the world, Americans would be among the most long-lived.

Such is not the case. In 2000, researcher Stephen Bezruchka forcefully called our attention to the "disgracefully poor" health of our citizens—and our national ranking of twenty-fifth in life expectancy—placing us "behind all the other rich countries and even a few poor ones."[10] A more recent study corroborated Bezruchka's findings—placing us in the bottom third relative to life expectancy among industrialized nations.

Numerous scholars, however, have challenged the validity of life expectancy as measured from birth as a meaningful indicator of the quality of a nation's health services. They argue that there are too many confounding variables influencing this measure, including patients' ability to access care.

Based on this argument, it is now fashionable to consider life expectancy from age sixty-five forward—a time when, thanks to Medicare, virtually everyone in America possesses the insurance coverage required to gain access to the health care system. When measured in this manner, "U.S. life expectancy for both men and women at age sixty-five is above the Organisation for Economic Cooperation and Development (OECD) average but below what the top countries have achieved, particularly for women."[11] The OECD is among the most frequently cited sources of comparative research on global health.

AN OUNCE OF PREVENTION

Life expectancy is but one measure of the quality of care we receive. There are many more metrics, including the rate of preventable deaths in the United States—which, by definition, includes the level of chronic illness amenable to treatment.

Research has consistently shown that the rate of preventable deaths in the United States is exceptionally high. One study ranked the United States dead last among nineteen countries in number of preventable or avoidable deaths.[12] Tobacco is the leading cause of preventable death in America, where more than forty-three million Americans light up every day.[13]

Smoking is but one of the many factors contributing to the high level of chronic conditions afflicting our population. It is interesting to note that, despite the fact that other nations have even worse nicotine habits, "the United States had a much higher prevalence of nine of ten conditions, including cancer, heart disease, and stroke, in its population over age fifty."[14]

ROBBING THE CRADLE

Another critical measure of the adequacy of our health care system is infant mortality. Our infant mortality rate, as measured against other wealthy nations, is the highest in the world—a claim that should be nothing short of embarrassing for a country of our stature. According to the National Academy of Sciences, this problem has existed for decades. And our problem is not limited to infant mortality. Our population also experiences lower birth weights and higher mortality rates before the age of five than other developed nations.[15]

Recently released data suggests that this bleak situation is brightening. According to a study released in April 2013 by the National Center for Health Statistics, infant mortality rates in the United States declined 12 percent between 2005 and 2011.[16] The greatest reduction in infant mortality was among non-Hispanic, black women. Improvement could be seen in four out of the five major causative factors of infant mortality.

But before we are too quick to celebrate, bear in mind that this substantive change in infant mortality means that the U.S. ranking among thirty industrialized nations moved from twenty-eighth to twenty-seventh.[17] That's hardly worth bragging about.

STILL UNCONVINCED?

If you are still plagued by doubts as to the validity of these damning assertions, consider the following excerpt from a report published in 2012 by the National Academy of Sciences. "The United States," they say, "is among the wealthiest nations in the world, but it is far from the healthiest. Although life expectancy and survival rates in the United States have improved dramatically over the past century, Americans live shorter lives and experience more injuries and illnesses than people in other high-income countries. A growing body of research is calling attention to this problem, with a 2011 report by the National Research Council confirming a large and rising international 'mortality' gap among adults age fifty and older."[18]

Is there any good news amid the doom? One might argue yes, based on our outcomes in treating cancer.

In 1971, President Nixon declared war on cancer. Though the disease remains a scourge with only modest progress made toward cures, the United States appears to be maintaining a leadership position in this battle. Cancer survival rates are generally better in the United States than in other countries. In fact, for patients afflicted with prostate, breast, colon, lung, and rectal cancer, the best chances for survival are in the United States.[19] Furthermore, "U.S. survival rates were also among the highest for melanoma (fourth), uterine (second), and ovarian (fifth) cancer, cervical cancer (sixth), Hodgkin's disease (third), and non-Hodgkin's lymphoma (fourth)."[20]

Though this may appear to be the silver lining in an otherwise dismal assessment of our health care system's performance, such rays of hope may have limited validity. There are many factors that influence cancer survival rates beyond the quality, availability, and accessibility of treatment options. Chief among them is the correlation among screening rates, early detection, and survival. As we will shortly see, the United States is aggressive in its screening behaviors—with the upside being additional survival rates and the downside being the potential for unnecessary, expensive, and potentially debilitating treatments.

The preponderance of evidence leads to the inexorable conclusion that Americans receive substandard care. In addition to its glaring flaws, it is also the most expensive health care in the world.

THE WORLD'S MOST EXPENSIVE CARE

I remember when a bottle of soda pop cost a dime. It came in an icy cold glass bottle with a cork-lined cap. Over time, the bottle and cap gave way to a can, and the price rose to a quarter, then half a dollar, and even a buck. But what if that soda had risen to twenty dollars? Would there have been a public outcry? At what point do we decide that the rate of cost escalation for an item or an industry is absolutely out of control?

There's a fitting irony to the fact that health care costs were first "officially" analyzed and recorded in 1929,[21] when the economy tumbled and the stock market crashed. Over the next two decades, prices remained relatively stable and consumed approximately 4 percent of the nation's gross domestic product (GDP).[22] Then all hell began to break lose. In 1950, health care costs were a "meager" $12.7 billion.[23] Three generations later, in 2012, those costs had risen to $2.6 trillion. That's more than a two-hundred-fold increase in the nation's health care bill! Based on that same 20,000 percent increase in price, our proverbial bottle of Coca-Cola would now cost twenty bucks!

Today, health care purchases consume more and more of every dollar we spend. The nation's health care bill has risen from 4.4 percent of

GDP in 1950 to nearly 18 percent in 2012. If you are wondering how that compares to the spending levels of other industrialized nations, the next highest OECD country, the Netherlands, spent 12 percent of its GDP on health care.[24]

Before you conclude that our spending levels are merely a reflection of the size of our population, take a look at average per capita spending. In 2012, the United States spent $8,233 for each citizen. That's approximately $5,000 more per capita than the average expenditures among all thirty OECD nations.[25]

The lowest spending OECD nations (New Zealand and Japan) consume approximately $3,000 per capita in health care services. Japan achieves this remarkably low level of spending despite the fact that it actually uses a tremendous amount of health care resources per capita. It simply manages costs far better than the United States.[26]

Americans are awakening to the fact that we have a system whose costs are out of control, and journalists are sounding the warning Klaxon. In an article published in the *Atlantic* in 2013, "Why Is American Health Care So Ridiculously Expensive," author Derek Thompson opined that "the U.S. medical system is absurdly expensive. You know that already. But you probably didn't realize just how absurdly expensive it is compared to other countries."[27]

While consumers' overall confidence in U.S. health care may be unfaltering, their awareness of its escalating costs is growing, as was revealed by a series of focus groups funded by the Robert Wood Johnson Foundation. The research, conducted in four major American cities, explored consumer sensitivity to health care costs.

The unambiguous conclusion drawn by the researchers was that "Universally, participants were aware of the effects the rising cost of care had on their pocketbooks and the accelerating speed at which costs have risen in recent years. That said, they didn't know why costs are going up or how to decipher them."[28] Perhaps most alarming, based on the respondents' feedback, researchers further concluded that "across the board, there was a sense that participants were nearing the breaking point."[29]

Even a cursory review of articles written about health care costs over the past forty years suggests that we've been at or near "the breaking point" for decades.[30] The term conjures powerful images of a runaway train, but will the train ever truly derail? More importantly, why is our nation's health care bill so high, and what can we do about it?

WHERE OUR MONEY GOES

Our astronomically high national tab for health care is driven by many factors, not the least of which is the high price we pay for health care products and services. Let's begin by breaking down the bill.

For every health care dollar we spend, approximately 31 percent goes to hospital care. Twenty percent is spent on the professional services rendered by physicians and clinics, and 10 percent buys drugs. The remaining 30 percent is spread across a number of categories.[31]

If we dig even deeper, it's amazing what we uncover. Take hospital charges, for example. When compared to other developed nations, our hospital costs are almost 2.7 times greater ($19,319 versus OECD median costs of $7,180 per discharged patient). That helps explain why the United States had 54 percent as many hospital discharges as Germany and yet our health care tab was still 190 percent greater per capita than Germany's.[32]

We also hit pay dirt when we dig into the issue of pharmaceutical costs. U.S. pharmaceutical spending per capita was nearly $1,000 in 2010—two times the OECD median.[33] That's not terribly surprising in light of the fact that we pay more for the top thirty pharmaceuticals— nearly three times as much as New Zealanders and twice as much as people in the United Kingdom.[34]

The sad fact is that the difference between U.S. drug prices and the price for exactly the same drug in other countries can be staggering. In the United States, the average cost of Lipitor, a commonly prescribed drug to treat high cholesterol, was approximately $100 in 2012. It was $6 in New Zealand.[35] You don't have to travel halfway around the world to experience this phenomenon. Anyone who has traveled across the border to Mexico has seen many of our prescription drugs sold over the counter for pennies on the proverbial dollar.

In essence, Americans are subsidizing lower drug prices in every other corner of the world, allowing pharmaceutical manufacturers to nonetheless maintain their historically high levels of profitability by charging us more.

PATIENTS IN GLASS HOUSES SHOULDN'T CAST STONES

The data proves irrefutably that most industrialized countries have healthier populations based on numerous metrics and that they accomplish this feat while racking up a mere fraction of the U.S. health care bill.

There's no greater illustration of this phenomenon than Japan, one of the most prolific consumers of health care services on the planet. Its population visits physicians with more than three times the frequency of Americans, yet Japan's total health care bill, on a per capita basis, was only 37 percent of the U.S. per capita spend.[36] As a country long enamored of technology, it is not surprising to learn that Japan has nearly five times as many MRI units as the average OECD country, yet the cost per scan, and thus overall contribution to the nation's health care bill, is quite low.

Japan does a great job of controlling its costs—and often does so in innovative rather than Draconian ways. One example is its purchase of MRI units. Because this imaging modality is heavily utilized by its physicians, Japan's health care providers need to be able to deliver MRI services cost-effectively. They accomplished this goal by working hand-in-hand with major Japanese technology firms, such as Toshiba, to develop far less expensive MRI units than those deployed in the United States. Though somewhat less sophisticated, these units nonetheless provide clinically satisfactory images for physicians.[37]

Americans love to loathe the British health care system. Yet a side-by-side comparison of costs for common surgical procedures shows the United Kingdom to be far more cost-efficient: The average cost for an appendectomy in the United States is $13,851 versus $3,408 in the United Kingdom. A normal, vaginal delivery in the United States is $9,775 versus $2,641 in the United Kingdom. And a C-section costs in excess of $10,000 more in the United States than in the United Kingdom. Finally, the total cost for coronary-bypass surgery averaged $73,420 in the United States. In the United Kingdom, it cost $14,117. In France, it cost $22,844.[38] Every time we say derisive things about *socialized medicine*, the Brits are laughing all the way to the bank.

Technologically advanced procedures may show an even greater difference in price. Fifty years ago, a Swiss physician performed the first percutaneous transluminal coronary angioplasty (a minimally invasive procedure for opening up clogged arteries). Today the average cost of that procedure in Switzerland is $5,295. In the United States, the average cost is more than five times as much—$28,182.[39]

If you are wondering who's making all the money, the answer is everyone associated with health care delivery in the United States. I'm only being somewhat facetious, as we shall see in the remaining chapters of this book. For now, let's take a look at just physician fees.

PROFESSIONAL OR PROFITEER?

Medicine may be recognized as a noble profession across the globe, but nowhere is it more remunerative than in the United States, where physicians enjoy phenomenally strong earnings when compared to their international brethren, which translates into higher fees for American patients. Average physician fees in the United States for a routine office visit in 2012 were $95 versus $30 in Canada and France.[40]

Surgical specialists in the United States fare particularly well. Surgeons in the United States receive fees almost three times greater than their counterparts in Canada for hip-replacement surgery.[41] U.S. orthopedic surgeons make more than twice as much as their Canadian counterparts (with cost-of-living adjustments factored in). Most notably, American obstetricians were paid more than five times as much to deliver babies as their foreign counterparts in Canada and France in 2012.[42]

Most Americans don't mind paying more for a measurably better product or service. The question, again, is, Are we getting value for each of the 2.8 trillion dollars we spend annually? Not according to global-health researchers Docteur and Berenson, who state, "In light of the fact that the United States spends twice as much per person on health care as its peers, those who question the value for money obtained in U.S. health expenditures are on a firm footing."[43]

They are far from alone in their belief. Another powerful voice in this choir belongs to Arnold Relman, editor emeritus of the *New England Journal of Medicine*. Relman wrote, "Considering that we spend so much more on medical care than any other advanced country, we ought to expect health outcomes to be at least as good and our citizens ought to be at least as satisfied with the system. But we can claim neither."[44]

FIRST DO NO HARM

Health care and its physician stewards harm more than just our pocket-books. Despite admonitions to *do no harm*, Americans are at risk every time we encounter the health care system. In fact, it appears that we are at a significantly higher risk of danger than patients in other nations. Out of seven nations studied, the United States ranked last in terms of patient safety.[45] The Netherlands topped the list.

These safety issues should come as no surprise to those of us involved in the industry, for we've often witnessed them firsthand. Marty Makary, MD, a surgeon, author, and health policy professor at Johns Hopkins, commented that "As a surgeon who has worked in some of the best medical centers in the nation, I can testify that American medicine is spectacular in many ways. . . . Yet this same medical system routinely leaves surgical sponges inside patients, amputates the wrong limbs, and tolerates the overdosing of children because of sloppy handwriting."[46]

In 1999, headlines around the world shouted similar news based on a report released by the venerable Institute of Medicine (IOM). *To Err Is Human: Building a Safer Health System* systematically examined the safety of our nation's health care system. The most startling findings were based on two research studies—one conducted in Colorado and Utah, the other in New York. "The results of the study in Colorado and Utah imply that at least forty-four thousand Americans die each year as a result of medical errors. The results of the New York study suggest the number may be as high as ninety-eight thousand."[47] Based on this data, medical error was responsible for more deaths annually than car crashes, breast cancer, or AIDS.[48]

Beyond its toll of death and destruction, the IOM report also assigned an economic cost to medical error, estimating the "total national costs . . . of preventable adverse events . . . [at] between \$17 billion and \$29 billion, of which health care costs represent over one-half."[49]

Despite the IOM publication's clear intent to catalyze constructive change, initial reactions were similar, in many respects, to the stages a recently diagnosed cancer patient goes through. First there was denial, then anger. Eventually, the health care industry moved cautiously toward a seeming acceptance of the validity of the powerful accusations leveled against medicine.

As one would expect from the repentant, there were promises made to change the system. Hospitals established major quality-improvement initiatives. Billions of dollars flowed into health care information systems that promised to keep a watchful eye on care processes.

Yet the resulting improvements in safety have been modest at best. "In 2010, a Harvard study published in the prestigious *New England Journal of Medicine* reported a finding well-known to medical professionals: As many as 25 percent of all patients are harmed by medical mistakes. What's even less known to the public is that over the past ten years, error rates have not come down, despite numerous efforts to make medical care safer."[50]

EQUAL RIGHTS FOR ALL . . . EXCEPT WHEN IT COMES TO HEALTH CARE

A final measure to consider when challenging the myth of the superiority of American health care is its comparative availability, accessibility, and equity. We can accomplish this by asking two basic questions: (1) Are all segments of our society able to access quality, efficient, and effective care? and (2) does one's societal class or ethnicity affect one's ability to receive the right care?

Clear indicators of failure on this measure have existed for many years. The *World Health Report 2000*, published by World Health Organization, ranked the United States fifty-fourth among nations relative to "fairness of financial contributions" for health care.[51]

According to a survey funded by the Commonwealth Foundation, "The U.S. ranks a clear last on nearly all measures of equity. Americans with below-average incomes were much more likely than their counterparts in other countries to report not visiting a physician when sick, not getting a recommended test, treatment, or follow-up care, not filling a prescription, or not seeing a dentist when needed because of costs."[52]

This lack of equity, which has been a hallmark of American health care, makes a life-and-death difference for some patients. "Several years ago," noted Otis Brawley, chief medical officer for the American Cancer Society, "my research team at the American Cancer Society published data showing that people diagnosed with cancer who had no insurance or were insured through Medicaid were 1.6 times more likely to die in five years as those with private insurance."[53]

As the spouse of an oncologist, I find such information of particular interest. My wife spent the first twenty years of her practice in an indigent setting. When she would return home after an exhausting day's work, I listened attentively as Lori recounted stories of patients unable to afford the care they needed, unable to arrange transportation to receive life-saving treatments and lacking the social support that would help make difficult diagnoses more survivable.

Many of my wife's patients were African Americans, who suffer disproportionately from the inequity of our flawed health care system. Her patients were not the exception. The evidence, which has existed for decades, overwhelmingly supports a cultural bias that discriminates against African Americans, as well as Hispanics. George Lundberg, former editor of the *Journal of the American Medical Association*, described the systematic racial bias:

> In a 1991 *JAMA* editorial I asserted that our health care system is guilty of institutionalized racism. The people involved don't even know it's going on. They don't recognize it. The cultural bias against the African Americans is particularly distressing. Studies have shown that, even when blacks have insurance under Medicare, significantly fewer procedures are performed on them. The studies document that fewer procedures, fewer diagnostic tests, and fewer therapies are performed on black Medicare beneficiaries than on white Medicare beneficiaries under exactly the same presenting circumstances, whether it be cancer, heart disease, diabetes, or stroke. This is as true in Minnesota as it is in Mississippi.[54]

You don't have to take Lundberg's word for it. Check out the government's own Agency for Health Care Research and Quality (AHRQ) website.[55] There you will find some very interesting statistics regarding ethnic or racial inequities in health care, including the following:

- About 30 percent of Hispanic and 20 percent of black Americans lack a usual source of health care compared to less than 16 percent of whites.

- Hispanic children are nearly three times as likely as non-Hispanic white children to have no usual source of health care.
- African Americans and Hispanic Americans are far more likely to rely on hospitals or clinics for their usual source of care than are white Americans (16 and 13 percent, respectively, versus 8 percent).[56]

DIAGNOSIS AND TREATMENT

Race and ethnicity influence a patient's chance of receiving many specific procedures and treatments. Of nine hospital procedures investigated in one study, five were significantly less common among African American patients than among white patients; three of those five were also less common among Hispanics, and two were less common among Asian Americans. Other AHRQ-supported studies have revealed additional disparities in patient care for various conditions and care settings, including:

- *Heart disease.* "African Americans are 13 percent less likely to undergo coronary angioplasty and one-third less likely to undergo bypass surgery than are whites."[57]
- *Asthma.* "Among preschool children hospitalized for asthma, only 7 percent of black and 2 percent of Hispanic children, compared with 21 percent of white children, are prescribed routine medications to prevent future asthma-related hospitalizations."[58]
- *Breast cancer.* "The length of time between an abnormal screening mammogram and the follow-up diagnostic test to determine whether a woman has breast cancer is more than twice as long in Asian American, black, and Hispanic women as in white women."[59]
- *Human immunodeficiency virus (HIV) infection.* "African Americans with HIV infection are less likely to be on antiretroviral therapy, less likely to receive prophylaxis for Pneumocystis pneumonia, and less likely to be receiving protease inhibitors than other persons with HIV. An HIV-infection data-coordinating center, now under development, will allow researchers to compare contemporary data on HIV care to examine whether disparities in

care among groups are being addressed and to identify any new patterns in treatment that arise."[60]

- *Nursing-home care.* "Asian American, Hispanic, and African American residents of nursing homes are all far less likely than white residents to have sensory and communication aids, such as glasses and hearing aids. A new study of nursing-home care is developing measures of disparities in this care setting and their relationship to quality of care."[61]

Some of these issues undoubtedly relate to insurance coverage. It is hoped that some of the disparity will be addressed when an additional thirty-two million Americans presumably receive coverage under the Affordable Care Act (ACA), which will be discussed in more detail in a later chapter. For now, it is important to note that the ACA will likely not be the panacea to our problems of inequity. "Nevertheless," as posited in a *Forbes* article of May 28, 2013, "with more than 20 percent of the nation's black population uninsured, more than 30 percent of Hispanics uninsured, and a country still grappling with understanding and properly addressing disparities, just how far does the ACA take us?"[62]

WHY IS THE SYSTEM SO BROKEN?

We've examined how the outcomes, cost, safety, and equity of American health care differ from care in other nations, but we've not sought to understand why.

After spending thirty years working in the health care industry, at the risk of gross oversimplification, I believe there are three fundamental factors contributing to its dysfunction: (1) the fragmented manner in which we pay for care, (2) the lack of price controls, and (3) the changing culture of medicine.

A FRAGMENTED PAYMENT SYSTEM WITH NO BRAKES

The United States has the most complicated system in the world for insuring its population and paying its national health care bill. It is a complex aggregation that includes federal plans, such as Medicare, state-driven plans, such as Medicaid, and a host of private insurers that operate as both for-profit and not-for-profit entities. The nongovernmental plans are far from uniform. Each plan may have a significantly different contractual arrangement with each provider in its network. The rates paid by an insurer to the medical-care practitioner will vary from patient to patient depending on the nuances of the patient's plan. So, too, will they vary by procedure from hospital to hospital.

This fragmentation and complexity results in dramatically higher administrative costs within our system, which contribute to our overall soaring health care bill. The United States leads all other industrialized countries in the share of national health care expenditures devoted to insurance administration. "The McKinsey Global Institute estimates that the U.S. spends $91 billion more a year on health insurance administrative costs than it should, given its size and wealth."[63] Arnold Relman, editor emeritus of the *New England Journal of Medicine*, believes that the United States "is unique in this regard." He says,

> We obviously pay dearly for the *privilege*: Other countries (for example, the United Kingdom, Germany, France, and Sweden) had universal, publicly supervised health insurance systems in place before, or soon after, the postwar technology revolution in medical care began. Unlike the fragmented and decentralized U.S. system, these public plans prohibit or discourage private enterprise from gaining more than a marginal position in their health care systems, and they usually regulate the prices paid to doctors and hospitals. The strong incentives to commercialization that were unopposed in the United States were essentially blocked by the prior existence of national health programs in these countries.[64]

Though any attempt to control prices brings outcries of "socialized medicine," other countries' insistence on price controls have helped keep the brakes on otherwise runaway costs. Our free-market beliefs and unbridled entrepreneurism are coming at a very high price—one that ultimately will be shouldered by you and me.

A CULTURE OF GREED

We have vested the medical community with the cultural authority to oversee our health care system and manage our health. For the first half of the twentieth century, physicians seemed to view this trust as sacred and worked toward the betterment of health care—at a patient level as well as a system level. Then things began to change.

First, the supply of physicians grew dramatically, as did the rate of specialization within the medical profession. "Since 1965," Relman has noted, "the number of physicians has grown four times faster than the population: 160 percent for physician growth versus 36 percent for population growth. In 1960 there were 142 physicians per 100,000 populations; now there are 282."[65]

At the same time, empowered by tremendous technological advances, medicine moved from being a profession built upon the quality and longevity of a trusting patient/physician relationship to a technocracy in which physicians armed with increasingly specialized knowledge and access to sophisticated treatment modalities intervene on "cases."

As a result, once driven by a combination of altruism and a fervor for harnessing scientific knowledge for the benefit of society, medicine has been increasingly replaced by entrepreneurism and greed. This factor is the most insidious of all and applies not only to a segment of the physician population but to many other stakeholders within the health care delivery system. Unfortunately, our trusted agents in health care have not stopped the avarice that increasingly defines our system.

In a beautifully worded editorial appearing in the *Annals of Internal Medicine* on March 15, 1996, Christine Cassell, MD, reminds us that "medicine is, at its center, a moral enterprise grounded in a covenant of trust. Today this covenant of trust is significantly threatened. From within there is growing legitimization of the physician's materialistic self-interest; from without, for-profit forces press the physician into the role of commercial agent to enhance the profitability of health care organizations."[66]

Cassell goes on to warn that "physicians, as physicians, are not, and must never be, commercial entrepreneurs, gate closers, or agents of fiscal policy that runs counter to trust. Any defection from primacy of the patient's well-being places the patient at risk by treatment that may compromise quality of or access to medical care."[67]

If America is ever to boast of delivering the best health care in the world, the system will require transformational change. Patients can advocate for such change, and should, but ultimately it is physicians who must be the architects of change.

WHAT YOU CAN DO TO PROTECT YOUR HEALTH

Congratulations—you've taken the first step on a very important journey: You've opened your eyes to the reality of American medicine and perhaps challenged some of the beliefs you once held. Removing the blinders is the first step on our journey together. As you proceed and your knowledge of the health system increases, so, too, will the breadth and depth of action you can take to improve the care you and your family receive.

MYTH 2
"SHOPPING FOR HEALTH CARE IS LIKE SHOPPING FOR A CAR; YOU BASE YOUR DECISIONS ON GOOD INFORMATION"

A propensity for heart disease was hard-wired into my mother's genes. Her father had died of a heart attack, and physicians had long warned my mother that she could suffer a similar fate. So it came as no surprise when one quiet afternoon she was suddenly gripped with overwhelming chest pain. But before the calamity could turn into a tragedy, my father summoned paramedics, who whisked my mother off to a nearby ER.

Minutes after crossing the threshold of the ER, one nurse was attaching the leads of an EKG to my mother's chest while another drew a blood sample. The EKG tracings, coupled with subtle indicators in her blood, provided clear evidence of a heart under siege. My mother was then handed off to cardiologists for an additional diagnostic workup so an appropriate treatment plan could be constructed rapidly.

A cardiac catheterization revealed numerous blockages in the major blood vessels flowing to my mother's heart. Atherosclerosis, or heart disease, had caused the occlusions. Without the appropriate intervention, the physicians told us, another heart attack was imminent. At the time, in the late eighties, the preferred treatment for my mother's condition was coronary artery–bypass surgery or "open-heart surgery," so we went shopping for a surgeon.

After several weeks of due diligence, we selected a physician to interview. The doctor we met with had a reputation for being the best cardi-

ovascular surgeon in the city. When I asked this highly respected sur-
geon if I could see his risk-adjusted mortality data for comparable pro-
cedures, he laughed and said, "You've got to be kidding." I was deadly
serious. I wanted to know his track record—how his patients fared
when compared to thousands of other patients undergoing similar pro-
cedures across the nation.

It was clear he wasn't asked this question with any regularity, but,
much to his credit, the doctor provided me with the information I
needed to feel completely confident about placing my mother's health,
and possibly her life, in his hands. My faith proved well placed, since
not only did my mother come through the surgery with flying colors but
she significantly outlived her prognosis, enjoying a bountiful life.

I was fortunate to have enough knowledge of the industry to help our
family find the best resources to care for my mother. But what about the
average American—how would they discern between a great surgeon
and one with an aberrantly high death rate among his or her patients?

There are no savvier consumers than Americans. Yet when it comes to
the most important purchase decisions we make—health care—we
don't know where to begin. Unlike other markets in which an understanding of comparative quality, costs, and value-driven decisions,
health care represents the pinnacle of blind trust.

Think, for a moment, about the last major purchase you made. Perhaps it was a car or a washer/dryer or even a house. If you are like most
Americans, you did your homework. You thought carefully about your
needs, researched all available options, contemplated the value you
would receive, and finally made a decision. After all, it would be a
decision that you would presumably live with for some time.

Yet how much thought do you give to major health care decisions?
How did you decide on your family doctor? How do you know that the
specialist your doctor recommends is the best available? When you
require treatment, how do you discern whether you've gotten all the
options in an objective fashion that allows you to make intelligent decisions regarding the benefits and risk?

And what about your hospital? Do you really know how it compares
to other facilities, or do you take the promises it makes in advertisements to be the gospel? You probably know how your car ranks in terms

of reliability or safety. Yet most Americans don't have a clue about the relative ranking of their hospital of choice.

Nor do they understand its costs. Private or government insurance pays the freight for most care, insulating the average person from the full burden of our inordinately expensive health care. Employers then generously offset much of the cost of insurance, which further isolates us from the direct impact of health care costs.

This separation of the patient from payer can significantly influence consumer behavior. When it's not their money, consumers may be markedly less demanding in seeking out information on comparative value. It's common to hear consumers say, "It's not coming out of my pocket, so why should I care?"

While beneficial to our pocketbooks, this arrangement may not be beneficial to our health. That's because the interests of the consumer or recipient of care and the purchaser—oftentimes the employer—may not be in alignment. While employers may have a wealth of information about the cost differential for health benefit plans based on various tiers of benefits or selection of specific provider networks,[1] these employers are often lacking comparative cost, quality, safety, and outcomes data for the providers in their networks. Their focus historically has been on cost containment, though that is slowly changing.

Since the economic power within health care is vested in the purchaser, not the patient, providers feel no particular obligation to provide transparent information that would allow patients to make smart comparisons on cost, quality, safety, and outcomes.

Think about it: Have you ever seen a price list for health care services? Sure, you know all about copays, but what about the real cost of care from your providers and how it compares to the charges of others? You might be surprised at the level of variance.

A cursory look at two common surgical procedures speaks volumes. The average charges for an appendectomy have been shown to vary from $2,000 to $180,000. Though not as dramatic, charges associated with hip surgery showed a ten-fold variation, ranging from $10,000 to as high as $100,000 (we will discuss how such variability in charges is possible in chapter 6).[2] Similar variance can be found in the costs of diagnostic tests. When charges associated with CT scans were compared across forty-nine metro markets, there was a 500 percent variance from the lowest to highest market. An even more dramatic variation in charges was found when blood cholesterol tests were analyzed; there was a twenty-fold variation in charges.[3]

WHAT YOU DON'T KNOW ABOUT HEALTH CARE MIGHT SURPRISE YOU

As we will see in detail in chapter 4, "these huge variations in price and quality occur not just across the country but across states, cities, and even among doctors practicing at the same hospital."[4] In other industries, such variation leads to the failure of those companies that either provide inferior products and services or charge uncompetitive pricing. These markets are self-regulating based on market dynamics. Why is health care an aberration?

WHAT'S THE MATTER WITH HEALTH CARE? WHY HEALTH CARE DOES NOT BEHAVE LIKE A MARKET

Markets are driven by the exchange of perceived value—with *value* being the buyer's perception of the comparative quality, cost, service, brand appeal, or other measures deemed important when considering a product. The more a buyer's perceptions are supported by objective, trustworthy information, the greater his or her confidence in making an intelligent purchase decision. Regardless of the specific criteria used to make a decision, consumers take comfort in the belief that their dollars are being well spent.

That's all fine and good when comparing cars, but in health care much of the data needed in making an informed decision either does not exist or is inaccessible to consumers. Even the most tenacious consumer who is doggedly determined to differentiate between providers based on comparative-value metrics may come up empty-handed. Even if they are fortunate enough to locate comparative data, they've only won half the battle. The next challenge is to properly interpret it so that it becomes useful.

There are additional challenges beyond the separation of the purchaser of care from the recipient of care coupled with the lack of actionable information regarding price, quality, and safety data. People purchase health care episodically and must often make decisions with great urgency rather than after contemplation. Whenever possible, we need to slow down and take whatever time is appropriate to understand our condition and intelligently explore our options.

THE COMPLEXITY OF HEALTH CARE

Medicine is horrifically complex. Like many other disciplines, it is enshrouded in a unique language that obscures its interpretation by lay consumers. Furthermore, there is still an "art and science" to medicine. Certain aspects of care can be quantified, while others are more elusive.

For transparency initiatives to be effective, there would need to be consensus about the criteria on which value-based decision making could be predicated. There would also need to be alignment between the patients and purchasers of care regarding the importance of having and acting on such information.

Even if they were provided with scientifically valid information, it would be difficult for consumers to understand the implications of much of the information—possibly causing them to come to erroneous conclusions or make improper decisions. Whether referring to cost or quality, the data must be user-friendly, according to the Institute of Medicine. "Consumer responsiveness to price," they say, "requires price data that are meaningful to them. Effective quality reporting needs to reflect different consumer abilities to understand and use information."[5]

Consumers can be confused not only by the terminology but also by the breadth and depth of data presented to them. Damman et al. found that "it is known that people can only process about six pieces of information at time and are easily overwhelmed by information. Therefore, providing all available information is not the most effective way to stimulate informed choices."[6]

THE LACK OF A TRUSTED RESOURCE FOR COMPARATIVE HEALTH CARE INFORMATION

Dependable resources need to be available to help consumers interpret health care information. For years, consumer health care advocates have bemoaned, If only there were a "Consumer Reports" of health care that allowed each of us to make rapid, smart decisions before any encounter with the health care system! *Consumer Reports (CR)* has responded, but its early efforts are in need of further refinement. Their "Health Ratings Center, formed in 2008, has published ratings on drugs, hospitals, health insurance, doctors, and diseases and preventive services. The popular consumer-products organization moved into health care to 'level the playing field' for everyday citizens who are inundated with ads and promotions, rather than facts, said John Santa, MD, director of the center."[7]

Consumer Reports' reviews and comparisons work for products and services that obey the traditional rules of a market-driven economy. Unfortunately, as we've demonstrated, health care is an aberration. Even so, the organization continues to labor to address the need for a trusted health care-information site for consumers.

In July 2013, *Consumer Reports* published "Your Safer-Surgery Survival Guide: Our Ratings of 2,463 U.S. Hospitals Can Help You Find the Right One." The article begins by alerting the reader to the high rate of surgical complications in American hospitals (stated to be as much as 30 percent). The authors then debunk some common consumer perceptions. They find that:

- Not all hospitals are created equal. In fact, hospitals vary widely in their surgical outcomes.
- Academic medical centers were generally poorer performers in *CR*'s analysis of surgical outcomes.
- A strong brand was no assurance of a positive outcome, citing Massachusetts General Hospital as an example—indicating that, despite its top, overall rating among American hospitals (according to *U.S. News and World Report*), it fared poorly on *CR*'s surgery measures.[8]

Online subscribers to *Consumer Reports* can find the top- and bottom-rated hospitals for various procedures broken out geographically at the *CR* website.[9]

What about other information sites? Should trusted consumer-information sites that survey other industries enter the health care arena? Likely contenders would include companies such as Angie's List, which currently provides limited reviews of providers, as well as TripAdvisor (one can envision a "HealthAdvisor").

The danger with sites that provide consumer reviews is the anecdotal nature of the information. Consumer impressions of quality may be fine when hiring a plumber or selecting a hotel for your family vacation but not when selecting a neurosurgeon. Patients may have found a provider charming—leading to a very high rating on a site—while the doctor's social skills may be a clever cover-up for a profound deficit in clinical skills. Those of us immersed in the industry know that bedside manner, while a highly valued skill, has no correlation to clinical competency.

There are sites that provide trustworthy information. Top among them are governmentally sponsored sites. Health plan sites may also contain valuable comparative information. Ironically, "the least trusted sources of information are health plans and government agencies—with only about one in twenty trusting those sources of information. Yet health plans and government agencies are far more likely to be able to assemble the required information."[10]

The bottom line is that, unlike the automobile industry, where a consumer can easily compare cost and quality between models, it is a far greater challenge in the murky world of health care.

BEWARE IMPOSTERS

A cadre of for-profit organizations has stepped in to capitalize on this void in information by ranking hospitals' performances across multiple clinical disciplines, such as heart care. Their rankings purportedly allow consumers to differentiate easily between providers of care, leading to value-driven decisions.

One such organization assigns a star ranking to hospitals, with five stars representing "best-of-class" performance. After bestowing the accolade, this vendor will magnanimously grant a license to the hospital to promote its star rating for a hefty fee. The fact that the hospital has purchased the promoted accolade is opaque to the consumer. So, too, are the details behind the methodology to assess performance and award the ratings.

There are other major players in the arena of purchased accolades. Though the variables on which vendors measure hospital quality differ, their methods are similar in that they bestow an accolade and then demand payment for its promotion.

These organizations are pervasive. In a four-week period, while serving as a senior vice president in a ten-hospital system, I was presented with the "opportunity" to purchase several such accolades for our hospitals. The cost to do so would have been hundreds of thousands of dollars. I declined the opportunity based on my conviction that it would only contribute to the further misinformation in an already confused marketplace.

MARKETING MISINFORMATION

A tremendous void of information is troubling enough. Misinformation designed to influence the uninformed consumer further exacerbates the problem, rendering intelligent decision making a Herculean challenge for consumers. Hospital marketing departments then add insult to injury by spending millions of dollars on exaggerated claims and erroneous assertions.

One example is hospitals' use of the designation *Center of Excellence*. Innumerable hospitals promote their "Centers of Excellence" in virtually every domain of clinical care.

Humana coined this term decades ago, and hospital marketers across the nation quickly latched on to it as an easy way of conveying a unique standard of care. I must confess that, as an early health care marketer in the 1980s, I, too, was guilty of this sin. The term became so ubiquitous over time as to render it meaningless. Whether it was a hospital with a robust cardiovascular program deeply staffed by highly trained specialists or a community hospital with a single "expert," each became a self-proclaimed *Center of Excellence*. It was the patient's job to exercise caveat emptor.

At times, these exaggerated claims of expertise cross the line from merely deceptive to outright egregious. A great example can be seen in the advertising for a community hospital in a Southeastern city.

The hospital launched an advertising campaign that proudly announced its expertise in the esoteric field of deep-brain stimulation—a delicate brain surgery in which a surgeon inserts electrodes into selected regions of the brain to ameliorate conditions ranging from seizures to intractable depression. This procedure has traditionally been the domain of major academic medical centers. In this case, the hospital bore no similarity to an "academic medical center." Rather, it had a single neurosurgeon who performed the procedures, and his training consisted of a weekend course.

Less insidious but nonetheless deceptive is advertising sponsored by certain National Cancer Institute–designated Community Cancer Centers. Some of these NCI centers have led consumers to the erroneous conclusion that the NCI designation signifies better or more advanced care. In reality, the NCI Community Cancer Center designation has precious little to do with the quality of care delivered. In fact, there is only one care-related question asked of applicants by the NCI: *Are 15 percent or more of your patients placed on clinical trials?* [11]

A second sin committed by these facilities—according to the American Cancer Society's chief medical officer, Otis Brawley, MD—is claiming that their patients fare better by virtue of the fact that the hospital is NCI designated. Says Brawley, "I'm very concerned about oncology centers that are bragging about survival rates. Most of them brag that people travel long distances to get to their facility. Well, only healthier people travel, so you have a huge selection bias for people who are going to live longer. It's not that the place makes people healthier." [12]

FLYING BLIND

So how do consumers make decisions regarding their health? Many of us predicate our conclusions on blind trust or the advice of well-wishing friends or family. Whether we get the care we need is a crapshoot.

Consumers, in general, also defer heavily to their physicians when it comes to making health care decisions, as was revealed by participants in a research study funded by the Commonwealth Foundation. Those participants stated that they prefer that their physicians tell them what to do. For example, one said, "Doctors shouldn't leave it up to you. He's the doctor."[13] Patients also rely on the doctor when they need to see a specialist: "Consumers rely on their physicians to make astute referrals, but the research reveals that 64 percent of physicians either rarely or never have quality-of-care data available when making a referral."[14]

Ideally, we should be able to defer to our physicians' judgments and recommendations regarding health care purchase decisions, but we will uncover the dangers inherent in this strategy shortly.

These are some of the reasons why it is oxymoronic to refer to health care as "market-driven." Unlike every other category of consumer goods and services, consumers can neither judge the relative quality and value of services they receive nor choose to support the most efficient and effective providers. As Collins et al. stated succinctly, "patients are in the weakest position to demand greater quality and efficiency."[15]

REMOVING THE BLINDERS BY ACHIEVING TRANSPARENCY

health care organizations bandy about the term *transparency*—using it to suggest an air of openness and disclosure about their performance and cost data. They have made repeated pledges to be more transparent. Unfortunately, they have been painfully slow in making good on their promises, causing the Institute of Medicine to observe that "a serious commitment to transparency means that we will strive to provide consumers with a comprehensive price and cost analysis, including effectiveness, adverse events, administration, and the impact of individual references relative to convenience and access."[16] Apparently this prestigious scientific body agrees that providers are not taking transparency seriously.

The absence of data is not merely a sin of omission. The health care industry has done a magnificent job of methodically shielding us from this vital information on which we could make value-based decisions regarding our health care. The providers simply don't want us to have the data: "A Commonwealth Fund National Survey of Physicians and Quality Care revealed that 69 percent of physicians were opposed to sharing quality-of-care data with the public. Forty percent of these physicians would not even allow their patients to be privy to such information."[17]

It's not just the doctors. Hospital executives want to be certain that any type of damaging information never appears on your radar screen. The 2003 Commonwealth Fund International Health Policy Survey of Hospital Executives revealed that hospital CEOs in the United States were significantly more opposed to public disclosure of medical error rates, hospital-acquired infection rates, patient satisfaction ratings, and average waiting times than CEOs in four economically advanced countries.[18]

DATA BEHIND CLOSED DOORS

Although you may not be able to access it, hospitals are nonetheless amassing a wealth of data on key quality variables. Federal mandates are partly responsible, though progressive hospitals interested in quality improvement are collecting data proactively. Some of the most important and potentially powerful data in terms of providing a window into the meaningful differences in quality between providers includes

- iatrogenic events,
- expected versus experienced mortality rates,
- sentinel events (in which the life of the patient has been threatened),
- surgical-infection rates,
- unscheduled returns to the operating room,
- readmission rates (which are now becoming publicly available), and
- punitive actions or sanctions imposed on physicians by their peers.

Don't be put off by the unfamiliarity of the terms. Though you may need some assistance with translation, you'll quickly grasp the significance of the measure. Take *iatrogenic events* for example, which, in plain English, translates into a hospital-acquired illness or injury.

Why do we care about something as esoteric sounding as "iatrogenic events"? We care because, by definition, an iatrogenic event is avoidable. Furthermore, it adds unnecessary costs and can even result in death or serious impairment. Imagine going to the hospital for a simple outpatient plastic-surgical procedure and having your surgeon accidentally ignite the oxygen you are breathing with an inadequately grounded electric cautery. It happened at one of my hospitals.

Iatrogenic events are not rare occurrences. Rather, they are daily events within the life of the American hospital. We generally only hear about them when they are egregious in nature, such as the amputation of the wrong limb, the overdosing of a patient, or the rapid spread of infection through a hospital. The media pay far less attention to the rate of falls in a given hospital, though such commonplace accidents can permanently impair an elderly patient who suffers a resulting hip fracture.

This paternalistic attitude and the resulting lack of information divulged to the public stymies market dynamics. Regardless of who is paying the health care bill, U.S. health care will never achieve true greatness without addressing the issue of transparency.

A BOLD EXPERIMENT

Mark Chassin, MD, observed this dramatic lack of transparency more than two decades ago. While serving as the health commissioner for New York State, Dr. Chassin became concerned about the perceived variability in outcomes for patients of open-heart surgery. Operating from the hypothesis that the death rates for this procedure varied dramatically between hospitals, Chassin embarked on a novel social experiment: he required all hospitals with open-heart-surgery programs in the state to report their outcomes. In an effort to minimize the argument that some patients were sicker than others, the hospital adjusted the data to account for patients' conditions and for demographic factors.

The data was stunning: "Among heart surgeons performing at least one hundred procedures a year, the risk-adjusted death rate ranged from zero to 11 percent. For those doing fewer than one hundred operations, by contrast, the death rates of individual surgeons ran as high as 82 percent for a doctor doing only nine cases."[19]

When the data was published, the outcry from providers was instantaneous. They were outraged at Chassin's gall in making public such potentially damaging information. They asserted that the outcomes data was highly suspect. In truth, the information was not only quite valid but also revelatory: "The first year that New York's hospitals were required to report heart-surgery rates, wide variation was found—the death rate by hospital ranged from 1 percent to 18 percent—confirming long-standing rumors that the quality of cardiac surgery was wildly variable among hospitals: Some places were outstanding while others were clearly flying by the seat of their pants."[20]

With their dirty laundry exposed, hospitals and their cardiac surgeons could either continue to cry foul or mobilize quickly to do damage control. Some hospitals exited the business, as did some of the worst-performing surgeons. Others focused on the underlying causes of their poor performance and worked assiduously to improve it. Mortality rates began to fall, and the deviation among hospitals' open-heart programs declined precipitously: "Statewide, deaths from heart surgery fell by 41 percent during the first four years of New York's public-reporting program and have continued to decrease ever since."[21]

New York was not the only state moving to address the questionable quality (as well as skyrocketing costs) produced by its hospitals and physicians. In 1986, the governor and Legislature of Pennsylvania signed into law Act 89, forming the Pennsylvania Health Care Cost Containment Council (PHC4). The stated goal of the council was to reduce costs and improve the quality of health care services by providing information to the consumers and purchasers of care that would stimulate competition among providers. In essence, PHC4 sought to catalyze market-based reform through improved transparency.

Six years later, in 1992, PHC4 published *A Consumer's Guide to Coronary Artery Bypass Graft Surgery* (open-heart surgery)—providing consumers, purchasers, and providers a window into the comparative performance of hospitals and surgeons. With little effort, the average Pennsylvanian could now identify the optimal combination of hospitals and surgeons to produce the best outcomes (as measured by mortality) at the least cost.

As in New York, the publication of the data had a powerful impact on the market. Providers scrambled to clean up their acts so as not to be the statistical outlier. The result: "Overall patient mortality rates dropped 22 percent from 1991 to 1995, and hospital charges for the procedure decreased for the first time since the state began reporting data in 1992."[22]

Twenty years later, the council's work continues, thanks to an extension of its charter by the legislature in 2009. Today its stated mission is to "restrain costs by stimulating competition in the health care market by giving (1) comparative information about the most efficient and effective health care providers to individual consumers and group purchasers of health services and (2) information health care providers can use to identify opportunities to contain costs and improve the quality of care they provide."[23]

From the more than 4.5 million patient records it collects annually, it distills information that should be highly beneficial to the marketplace. Whether consumers, purchasers, and providers have optimally leveraged this information to improve quality and outcomes has not been well quantified.

Neither of these two states' efforts would have gotten off the ground without the development of risk-adjustment algorithms. These mathematical formulas, which are used in an effort to level the playing field by accounting for the severity of a patient's condition (as well as other factors), squelched attempts by disgruntled physicians to invalidate research based on claims that their patients were "sicker."

Before the advent of this methodology, providers were quick to claim that their patients were different. Though the formulas themselves were often the target of criticism, the risk-adjustment methodology nonetheless became an essential tool for studying clinical outcomes among a diverse patient population while negating charges of inequity by providers.

A CRITICAL LESSON FROM THE EARLY PIONEERS: VOLUME EQUALS QUALITY

One critical finding from both New York and Pennsylvania was the correlation between volume and outcome. The data revealed that those hospitals and surgeons with higher volumes were significantly more likely to produce better outcomes and lower mortality than their lower-volume peers. The importance of this finding is its simplicity. Volume became an easy proxy for quality in the minds of consumers, who were otherwise ill-prepared to evaluate hospitals and surgeons.

Another important finding was the lack of correlation between quality and cost. Far from being a guarantee of higher quality, greater costs were often associated with inferior outcomes. It turned out that some high-volume hospitals had so refined and standardized their clinical processes that they were able to deliver a superior product at a lower cost.

With such an auspicious start, the transparency movement seemed destined to reshape the American health care landscape and truly catalyze market-driven reform. Health care activists were quick to proclaim that society was rapidly moving toward a day when health care would no longer be a blind purchase and a "Consumer Reports" would guide consumers' health care decisions.

Many of us within the industry hoped that as consumers coupled this newly available outcomes data with comparative cost information they would see, at a glance, how their area hospitals compared in value. Unfortunately, after these initial successes, transparency sputtered and sparked, never burning as brightly again.

Today there is certainly more information publicly available regarding provider performance, but the deficits far outweigh the gains made over twenty-five years. There are numerous reasons for the lack of transparency, beginning with the difficulty of establishing what data to collect and why.

CURRENT STATUS OF STATE INITIATIVES

Despite a seemingly auspicious beginning, state-transparency initiatives have been slow to advance over the past two decades. While some lack of momentum is understandable due to the difficulty in quantifying variations in quality, there are few such restrictions on quantifying variations in price. Yet when two advocacy groups that are both committed to greater transparency and price reformation jointly issued a report card rating the performance of states' initiatives, twenty-nine states received a failing grade followed by seven D grades "for policies that keep patients and their families in the dark on prices."[24]

Did any state fare well on this measure? Only two states scored an A—Massachusetts and New Hampshire—and that was by grading on the curve: "No state has implemented laws that meet all of our criteria."[25]

Uwe Reinhardt, one of the nation's leading health care economists, concludes that "it is truly remarkable that few state governments have made any effort to provide their residents with greater price transparency in health care, as well they could and should."[26]

MEASURING THE MEANINGFUL

The core measure of outcome in these early experiments was mortality, which appeared to be logical when dealing with life-and-death procedures in which mortality was a statistically significant reality. As a binary variable (*You survive or you perish*), it was easily understood by consumers. Furthermore, it possessed shock value, as patients awakened to the realization that their fate might be determined as much by the facility and/or surgeon they selected as by the nuances of their medical condition. It was certainly important to me when guiding my family on the selection of my mother's heart surgeon!

Mortality, however, is a crude measure in many ways. It gives us little insight into the quality or value delivered in less-acute services— such as maternity, where, fortunately, death is a rare aberration. As such, hospitals needed new measures to provide meaningful insight into the level of inexplicable variations in care and/or outcomes.

C-SECTION RATES RISE ALARMINGLY

In the case of maternity, one such measure is the rate of caesarean sections performed by a given provider or at a specific hospital. C-sections are an operation involving risk, albeit low, to mother and baby. They require longer recoveries and consume far more resources than "natural" childbirth.

When a baby is in distress, or other conditions threaten the health of mother and baby, a C-section can be a lifesaver. But how often is the intervention truly necessary? Over the past two decades, C-section rates have increased dramatically. The question is whether this increase is clinically justified.

The best-known recommended upper limit for C-sections is 15 percent, suggested by the World Health Organization (WHO)—a recommendation supported by two recent observation studies.[27]

C-section rates vary dramatically across obstetricians and their aligned hospitals. Intermountain Healthcare, a Salt Lake City–based health system known for its pioneering advancements in quality, utilization, and costs, maintains a low C-section rate relative to hospitals across the nation. Over a ten-year period, it reduced its C-section rate by 25 percent and also saved its payers of health care an estimated $50 million, according to an interview conducted by *Boston Globe* writer Deborah Kotz with its chief quality officer, Dr. Brent James.[28]

Mothers and their babies did not suffer as a result of this decline, according to Kotz's article, which went on to state that "the Intermountain hospital system, which handles thirty-four thousand deliveries a year, experienced no rise in death rates or serious complications in mothers or babies after putting its policies into effect."[29]

Intermountain Healthcare's experience in reducing and stabilizing the C-section rate is the exception in a nation afflicted by an epidemic of such procedures. A 2010 study by the National Center for Health Statistics provides the evidence:

> The Cesarean rate rose by 53 percent from 1996 to 2007, reaching 32 percent, the highest rate ever reported in the United States.
>
> Cesarean rates rose significantly in each state from 1996 to 2007. The magnitude of the increases varied. Six states (Colorado, Connecticut, Florida, Nevada, Rhode Island, and Washington) had increases of over 70 percent. In thirty-four states, Cesarean-delivery rates increased by 50 percent or more. In 2006, cesarean delivery was the most frequently performed surgical procedure in U.S. hospitals.[30]

Myriad factors contribute to the escalating rates of this procedure—from variations in socioeconomic status affecting the level of prenatal care given expectant mothers to a mother's increased age at the time of birth, both of which contribute to higher complication rates. Physician practice patterns certainly enter into the equation, as do consumer attitudes. If women believe that a C-section is a faster, safer path through the difficult and sometimes scary childbirth process, obstetricians may be glad to oblige.

The costs associated with these potentially unnecessary surgeries, when examined on a national basis, are astronomical. If one health system in Utah saved payers $50 million, imagine the savings that could be realized across the nation.

The "cure" for this problem begins by establishing evidence-based, accepted standards for the performance of a C-section and then helping consumers and physicians understand the importance of their adoption. Data from WHO suggests the need for radically fewer procedures.[31]

Childbirth and open-heart surgery represent the extremes in a "cradle to grave" health care system. What about all the other medical and surgical services delivered daily by hospitals and physicians? Are there meaningful metrics for assessing quality, value, and safety that could help direct our decision making?

THE DIFFICULTY OF ESTABLISHING HARD MEASURES FOR CLINICAL OUTCOME

Nothing beats hard facts when trying to make good decisions. Unfortunately, due to the dearth of publicly available, quantitative information, we also need subjective evaluations of clinical performance. Any surgeon will tell you that knowledge, judgment, and surgical dexterity are critical to positive outcomes, and there are no quantitative measures for these variables.

Any surgical nurse who has scrubbed in with a variety of surgeons will tell you that there is phenomenal variation in these dimensions across surgeons—resulting in markedly different outcomes. I've heard such nurses sing the praises of countless surgeons. I've also heard them remark, when no physician is within earshot, "I wouldn't take my dog to that doctor."

How does this variation affect your outcome? Sometimes the variation results in changes to length of stay, complication rates, or readmission—all of which are measureable. Sometimes, however, the variations in outcome are very difficult to assess.

Take, for instance, orthopedic procedures. How does a patient know whether they have experienced an optimal outcome? It may be by subjective assessment of the reduction in pain or improvements in range of motion. If patients use these measures, then the difference between the patient's expectations and their experience determines the outcome—hardly a scientifically, quantifiable metric.

Cancer surgeries represent an area where variation can take a huge toll in quality of life or life itself. One surgeon when confronted with a difficult colorectal cancer may elect to perform a life-changing colostomy (attaching an external bag to the abdomen to collect fecal matter), whereas another surgeon, operating under comparable conditions, is able to excise the tumor while sparing the patient the need to undergo the colostomy. This variation in approach may be more a factor of the surgeon's training and technical skills than the best interests of the patient. As patients, we presumably want our condition and health status to drive treatment decision, not the dexterity and skill of the surgeon.

Cancer surgeries can also be quite variable in terms of cosmetic results. Surgery for breast cancer represents a prime example of the degree of variability in cosmetic outcome. Some surgeons' results seem to suggest a lack of concern for the level of disfigurement caused by their intervention. This again raises the question of how one quantifies the variation in quality or outcome in such cases. It's not nearly as simple as looking at survival rates.

YOU CAN LEAD A HORSE TO WATER...

The publication of clinical and cost information resulted in some meaningful changes in New York and Pennsylvania—including elimination of poorly performing physicians who imperiled patients. The changes, however, were not due to consumers acting upon the potent information they were provided: "Studies fairly systematically find that public information on quality is not used by patients. New York and Pennsylvania were pioneers in publishing information on cardiac-surgery mortality by name of surgeon and hospital, yet few patients availed themselves of this information."[32]

If consumers did not drive change, who did act on the data? It was hospitals' CEOs, who were concerned about the negative public relations that might accrue to their program, as well as the contingent liability associated with knowingly maintaining a substandard program.

They worked quickly to weed out physicians who were failing to perform within the range of acceptable standards, while correcting other deficits in their programs.

Unfortunately, the willingness to act on powerful clinical data, by either consumers or health care leaders, may have dwindled, according to Alan Enthoven, a leading health care researcher and strategist:

> Two examples illustrate both consumers' and providers' indifference to the available data. First, the most high-profile [coronary-artery bypass graft] patient in the nation—former president Bill Clinton—chose to undergo this procedure at New York-Presbyterian Hospital/ Columbia University Medical Center in 2004, although this hospital ranked twenty-second in risk-adjusted CABG mortality rates among thirty-six hospitals performing the procedure in the state.
>
> In a more disappointing example, the Pennsylvania Health Care Cost Containment Council published a consumer guide to CABG surgery with risk-adjusted mortality data. In a random sample of 50 percent of Pennsylvania cardiologists, 87 percent said that the guide had little or no influence on their referral recommendations.[33]

The failure of physicians to consider this data was disappointing, particularly when one considers that researchers who examined the cost and outcomes for patients admitted to large Pennsylvania hospitals for acute myocardial infarction, or heart attack, found that the highest-costing hospital was more than four times as expensive (as measured by charges) than the hospital producing the lowest mortality rate.[34]

IS THE QUEST FOR MORE DATA MERELY A FIELD OF DREAMS?

Based on our findings, we must ask, *If we build it, will anyone come looking for the information?* Though consumers state that they want more information, when it is provided they fail to take advantage of it. Their failure to act may be more a symptom of their lack of awareness of the variability in cost, quality, safety, and accessibility of care, coupled with misperceptions about value, than a comment on their ambivalence. The results from a series or focus groups conducted by the Robert Woods Johnson Foundation seem to support this conclusion.

One major and consistent finding across the groups was that "participants repeatedly said they wanted to see a resource, or ask their doctor, to better understand what a particular test or procedure would cost before they agreed to it and wanted to comparison shop among providers when possible. . . . They were very interested in efforts to share information on price and quality."[35]

Consumers' ability to act on price and quality data may be encumbered by preconceptions that they possess: "Due to experience with other commercial goods and services, many consumers believe that cost is an indicator of provider quality and that 'you get with you pay for.' Thus, many consumers assume higher-cost hospitals or doctors' offices have more knowledge, experience, staff, and amenities or provide more specialized care."[36]

Peter Ubel, writing in the *Atlantic*, reinforced this point: "People assume the cost of a good or service tells them something about its quality."[37] Ubel went on to point out that "studies show that expensive pain pills reduce pain better than the same pills listed at lower price. Price, then, leads to a placebo effect."[38]

In another study, researchers examined consumers' willingness to accept marginally inferior clinical services if they were delivered at a greatly reduced cost. The scenarios varied "marginally in expected effectiveness but varied substantially in price."[39] All members had insurance coverage.

The researchers discovered that "the majority of participants were unwilling to consider costs when deciding between two nearly comparable options and generally resisted the less expensive, marginally inferior option," and the most frequently cited reasons for these attitudes included

- preference for the best care option, regardless of the costs involved;
- inexperience with making trade-offs between health and money;
- lack of interest in costs borne by society because of misunderstanding the way insurance works;
- lack of perceived personal responsibility; and
- disdain for insurance companies and the government.

"This preference for the best at any cost seemed to be a result of both participants' personal values—that their health is paramount—and their default assumptions about the relationship between care costs and quality."[40]

WHAT YOU CAN DO TO PROTECT YOUR HEALTH AND RECEIVE THE CARE YOU DESERVE

Now that we have stripped away some of health care's lustrous veneer and seen the level of variability in quality and cost among providers, how do we intelligently navigate the system to obtain value-driven care?

The first step is education. Though finding and interpreting comparative data may be an arduous task, we nonetheless need to undertake the process. One of our starting points is the Web. Remember, though, that the Web is about as regulated as the Wild West. Therefore, we need to be familiar with a number of rules of engagement before we begin our search to help ensure that we are accessing trustworthy information. When viewing a website, consider

- the objectivity of its sponsor,
- the potential biases in the data based on the site's perceived level of objectivity,
- the rigor of the methods used to analyze data,
- the timeliness and accuracy of the data, and
- the ease of interpreting and applying what you learn.

I'm not asking you to be an academic researcher, simply a curious consumer.

Our journey begins with key governmental websites, which help consumers differentiate between hospitals and physicians using the robust Medicare data set. Unfortunately, at the time of this writing, Centers for Medicare and Medicaid Services has "temporarily" suspended publication of key elements of this data—bowing to pressure from provider groups. If restored, the site has the power to provide easy and meaningful side-by-side comparisons of hospitals on such measures as hospital infection rates as well as relevant information about physicians.

A good place to start is with the federal government–sponsored Healthcare.gov, while the Centers for Medicare and Medicaid Services will provide comparable access.[41]

Consumers have been slow to avail themselves of such sites. Though the study is somewhat dated, a Kaiser Foundation survey conducted in 2008 found that a meager 8 percent of U.S. adults were familiar with the Medicare sites allowing hospital comparisons.[42]

Some state governments have also taken a leadership position in health care transparency. Among them is Florida, which allows consumers to access sophisticated but comprehensible comparative information about hospitals across the state.[43] The state of Massachusetts publishes similar data at MyHealthCareOptions®.[44]

As noted earlier, health plans may also be a valuable source of objective comparative information. Such plans have a strong incentive to steer their insured toward the most cost-effective care (though not necessarily the highest quality). UnitedHealthcare provides its insured members with a number of tools—including a price comparison tool.[45]

The *Consumer Reports* website was discussed earlier in this chapter. Though the information it contains is still somewhat limited, the integrity of the information is beyond reproach.

Major health care foundations can also be an invaluable and trustworthy source of information, though most have understandably shied away from direct physician-to-physician or hospital comparisons. Even so, these sites contain important guidance on issues critical to the informed health care consumer. Begin your investigation with these three superb sites—the Commonwealth Fund, the Robert Wood Johnson Foundation, and the Kaiser Family Foundation.[46]

There are a myriad of other foundations—some of which primarily focus on a limited geographic region but generally contain a wealth of information with applicability across all borders: California Health Care Foundation and California Endowment Foundation are two.[47]

There are also foundations that focus on singular diseases. The Caregiver Alliance publishes a listing of disease-specific foundations with accompanying descriptions and hot links to the sites.[48]

Finally, consumers may wish to explore commercial sites but should do so with their eyes wide open. One site worthy of your investigation is Healthcare Bluebook,[49] which purports to provide a "fair price to pay for a service or product when the patient is paying cash at the time of treatment. It represents a payment amount that many high-quality providers accept from insurance companies as payment in full, and it is usually less than the stated 'billed charges' amount."[50] Since pricing is a very complex issue in health care, one should approach any such provided information with caution.

I could go on ad infinitum listing websites for your perusal. And with each passing month the number of these sites will undoubtedly continue to expand

Despite the advances of the digital age, a great deal of important information is still to be found in books. You will be well served by reading voraciously about health care. Here's an initial reading list for your consideration:

> *Unaccountable: What Hospitals Won't Tell You and How Transparency Can Revolutionizes Health Care*, Marty Makary, MD
> *Demanding Medical Excellence*, Michael Millenson
> *The Last Well Person: How to Stay Well Despite the Health Care System*, Nortin M. Hadler, MD
> *A Second Opinion*, Arnold S. Relman, MD
> *To Err Is Human: Building a Safer Health Care System*, Institute of Medicine

Your next task in separating health care reality from fantasy regards advertising claims. Your job, should you choose to accept it, is to become an astute critic of such ads. This is not mission impossible but, rather, a relatively easy thing to do when guided by a few basic principles:

- Focus on the purely informational content of the ad—the facts associated with announcing the availability of newly expanded services, physicians who have joined the staff, or other incontrovertible facts. Such ads serve a purpose.
- View any claims that contain words such as *the only*, *the best*, *state-of-the-art*, and *the leader* as hyperbole or puffery. At the very least, demand proof in the form of facts supporting the assertion. This proof should be quantitative data that validates a claim (e.g., volume, outcomes, and costs).

- Completely ignore ads that talk about how much a hospital or physician clinic cares for you. That's their job. If they have to promise it in an ad, something is wrong.
- Do not be unduly swayed by testimonials. . . . They may represent a sample of one.
- Give no credence to celebrity endorsements. The actors are collecting huge fees to align their personal brands with those of your local hospital.
- Trust your gut. If an advertisement seems unbelievable, it probably is.

If you approach advertising as propaganda, you will be well on the road to being impervious to its pitch. Remember, there's often a grain (or more) of truth in propaganda, but it is spun and massaged in ways designed to manipulate you.

Because much of the information you receive about health care may occur while talking "over the fence" with your neighbor, it's important to put this in context. Your neighbor's opinion could be predicated on a great understanding of available providers or on nothing more than how the physician who treated her hemorrhoids made her feel. In other words, I would venture to bet that shared information, nine out of ten times, will be purely anecdotal.

If your neighbor is a physician or nurse, the quality of information may be slightly better. But it also may reflect strong biases rather than facts. So, factor all these comments from friends and family into your equation, but weight this grist more lightly.

EVEN WHEN ARMED WITH THE "RIGHT" INFORMATION, THERE WILL STILL BE OBSTACLES TO OVERCOME

Finally, it is important to remember that, even when armed with data, consumers do not always make logical decisions. After all, what could be more emotionally laden than important health care decisions? "Patients usually know much less about the diagnosis and treatment of their disease or injury than their doctors do," Arnold Relman writes. "As a consequence they cannot independently decide what medical services they want in the same way that consumers choose services in the usual market, shopping for what they want, at the prices they are willing to pay. The penalties for making a mistake in the health care market are usually higher than in others."[51]

MYTH 3
"MEDICAL INTERVENTIONS ARE BASED ON SCIENTIFIC EVIDENCE OF POSITIVE OUTCOMES REGARDING BEST PRACTICES; AS A RESULT, PATIENTS RECEIVE PRECISELY THE CARE THEY NEED"

Brandy and Keith Brown welcomed their baby daughter, Aspen, into the world with tears of joy. Their prayers had been answered—a healthy, beautiful, cherubic girl, who weighed in at seven pounds, eleven ounces. They couldn't wait to get Aspen home and begin their life together as a family.

The initial days and weeks blurred as everyone settled into a new routine. And though the early months were challenging, they were largely unremarkable. Aspen appeared to be developing right on schedule. But then things began to change. "At eight months, her motor skills seemed to be deteriorating. By her first birthday, she still wasn't crawling or talking."[1] Shortly thereafter, Brandy and Keith received devastating news. Aspen was diagnosed with Tay-Sachs—a genetic disease that was 100 percent fatal. Her life span, they were counseled, would be painfully brief.

When faced with such a diagnosis, parents will go to the "ends of the earth" to help their ailing child. Brandy and Keith Brown were no exception. Undaunted by what appeared to be a death sentence, they sought numerous medical opinions, but the answer was always the same—medicine had little or nothing to offer. Desperate to find a cure, they turned to Dr. Burton Feinerman.[2]

Dr. Feinerman had used a novel treatment involving stem cells in an attempt to repair damage to the brain of a boy from their town who had been involved in a serious accident.[3] Though he had never attempted to treat a patient afflicted with Tay-Sachs, Feinerman consented to the Browns' request to see Aspen and arranged for her treatment. Shortly thereafter, the family travelled to Peru in order for their daughter to receive stem cell injections.

Their precious baby daughter's life was in the hands of a physician in his early eighties with no formal training in stem cell research. Dr. Feinerman had spent the lion's share of his career practicing pediatric medicine in south Florida. Feinerman also provided "cosmetic dermatology" services to patients in Hawaii.[4]

When not providing potential miracle cures, Dr. Feinerman operates a medical practice in Florida "where he offers cell-repair treatments and hormone therapy to patients who want to look and feel younger."[5] A medical fountain of youth actually sounds relatively innocuous when compared to experimenting on children with unproven modalities of care that costs tens of thousands of dollars.

Feinerman's clinic sent hundreds of patients to his colleagues in Peru for stem cell injections. A few were afflicted with Tay-Sachs. According to his advertisements, "he can treat devastating and incurable diseases including Parkinson's, Alzheimer's, ALS, and Tay-Sachs."[6] All one needs is a pot of money and a willingness to get on a plane and travel to South America. Travel is required because there is no evidence supporting the safety or efficacy of the experimental treatments and thus they lack approval by the FDA.

Feinerman's stem cell "therapy" represents an extreme—the fringe of "medicine" that patients or their loved ones turn to when hope has vanished. He is but one of many physicians offering unproven and potentially dangerous modalities of care. Sometimes the treatment is an injection. For other physicians, it may be a device—such as the Rife machine, which purportedly cures cancer by using high-frequency energy.[7] When life ebbs, anything seems a better bet than sure death.

TRUST IN GOD, BUT FROM ALL OTHERS DEMAND PROOF

Modern medicine has pulled off a remarkable coup—it has convinced an unsuspecting public that the interventions delivered by its physicians are uniformly based on scientific evidence. That's why physicians such as Dr. Feinerman can practice with impunity.

The efficacy and safety of all therapeutic interventions fall somewhere along a continuum. At one extreme are those interventions whose safety and efficacy have been impeccably researched and documented; and at the other are unproven, unsafe treatments offered by physicians profiting from the despair of their patients. In between reside thousands of medical treatments whose relative efficacy and safety fall in the gray zone.

It's the gray area that is most concerning. In these unproven waters, physicians are able to offer a dizzying array of treatments with only anecdotal evidence of effectiveness.

If we are to protect patients by providing them with the "right" care and *only* the right care, I believe that there need to be five immutable laws governing medical interventions:

1. The intervention creates greater benefit to the restoration or promotion of health than harm (a Hippocratic admonition).
2. There is, at a bare minimum, some understanding of the mechanism by which the intervention is effective.
3. The efficacy and safety of the intervention, relative to other potential treatments, has been scientifically validated using proven methods, most notably rigorous, double-blind studies.
4. The patient is truly informed as to the benefits and risks associated with the intervention based on the data, as well as the alternatives.
5. The physician does not stand to profit disproportionately by selecting one treatment over another.

As I am not a physician, my bold assertion may unleash the wrath of physician critics emboldened by the audacity of a layperson to tread on such hallowed ground. So allow me to "borrow a page" from a Roundtable report published by the venerable Institute of Medicine (IOM) in 2007. "A core objective for the nation," it notes, "is achieving the best health outcome for every patient. This objective simply cannot be accomplished until we have better evidence on which to base health care decisions, as well as more effective application of the knowledge we have. Each is vitally important. We know, for example, that failure to deliver proven interventions is a substantial challenge to the quality of health care for Americans—and is a key concern of the IOM Roundtable on Evidence-Based Medicine."[8]

If you think about that for a brief moment, you quickly realize the fine veneer that separates the claims of medicine from the truth. If not based on solid scientific evidence, then what are many interventions predicated on? According to researchers at Dartmouth, "many diagnostic and therapeutic techniques are adopted or discarded on the basis of fashion or physicians' personal experience rather than on more reliable grounds."[9] I would add "greed" to this list of factors fostering adoption.

WHY IS MEDICINE RIFE WITH DELIVERY OF UNPROVEN, UNJUSTIFIED, INEFFICIENT, OR EXCESSIVE INTERVENTIONS?

What forces would be powerful enough to cause this fundamental abdication of scientific principles? There are four primary culprits.

Reason 1: The Cost and Complexity of Scientific Research

Medicine simply lacks the requisite infrastructure to validate treatment methods. There is no "centralized authority" vested with the power to conduct meaningful studies of the efficacy, safety, and efficiency of new therapeutic modalities, according to the American College of Physicians. As a result, the burden of proof falls on a hodgepodge of governmental, not-for-profit, and private entities. "This pluralistic system leads to large-scale duplication of efforts to provide evidence-based guidance to good medical practice."[10]

Even if there were a centralized authority, scientific research is anything but easy. The gold standard of scientific research in medicine is the double-blind study, which is designed to demonstrate the comparative effectiveness and safety of an intervention versus a placebo or alternative intervention. Its results are stated in terms of the statistical significance of the findings.

Such studies are difficult to design and even more difficult to implement. First, great thought must be given to the research method to both minimize confounding variables that may render such research invalid, as well as provide sufficient statistical "power" to give credence to the results. The design must be approved by an internal review board that sanctions the research method as being ethically and clinically appropriate.

Once the study is approved, participants who meet the research criteria must be recruited. Depending on the criteria for inclusion, the recruitment process may vary dramatically in its complexity and the time required. Because the validity of the research can be compromised by participants withdrawing prematurely from the process, consideration must be given to stemming attrition.

The actual research may require months, years, even decades to complete—particularly if the goal of the research is to show the relative efficacy of a treatment in ameliorating or preventing a condition or its recurrence. This is particularly true in cancer research, where recurrences may occur years after the initial presentation of the disease. That's why it is essential, in such research, to allow an appropriate interval of time to pass before drawing potentially inaccurate conclusions.

No wonder there is a dearth of comparative research that would help validate the appropriateness of many contemporary interventions. The one major exception to this rule is prescription pharmaceuticals, which are required by the Food and Drug Administration (FDA) to undergo vigorous comparative testing. Even here, however, there are numerous factors that may compromise the integrity of this research, as we will see in chapter 7.

So while vast sums of money are being allocated to the marketing of the latest and "greatest" medical advancements by manufacturers intent on ginning up sales, a mere pittance is going to the comparative research needed to justify their adoption. In 2007, the total U.S. investment in comparative-effectiveness research amounted to less than 0.1 percent of our nation's health care bill.[11]

Reason 2: The Pace of Technological Change and Expansion of Knowledge

There has been an explosion in the number of new treatment modalities coming to market, making the scientific validation of such treatments a daunting challenge: "From 1991 to 2003, the number of medical-device patents per year doubled, and biotechnology patents tripled. Between 1993 and 2003, there was an 80 percent increase in the number of prescriptions received by Americans. A recent review suggests that half or more of the growth in medical spending in recent years is attributable to change in technology."[12]

Just as there has been extraordinary growth in the rate of newly introduced medical technologies, there has been parallel growth in medical knowledge. A clear example can be seen in early genomic research that has already brought about a sea change in the way certain diseases, including cancer, are conceptualized.

Such knowledge, if properly harnessed, could ultimately catalyze transformational change in the diagnosis and treatment of a wide array of diseases and chronic conditions. But scientific discoveries must be vigorously validated. Then they must be incorporated into the corpus of knowledge that we call "medicine." Finally, the practitioners of medicine must be able to avail themselves of this knowledge in a timely fashion—and know how to use these new modalities correctly.

It all sounds so reasonable, but it requires phenomenal time and commitment on the part of doctors, who are already stressed by the need to increase productivity to offset reduced reimbursement for their services. How do physicians, whose incomes are governed by strict productivity standards established by their employers, balance their needs to earn good incomes against the time required to stay current on the state of the art in medicine?

That's the dilemma that many physicians face today. It is not a lack of desire to bolster their clinic knowledge and skills but a basic limitation of resources imposed by competing demands for time.

Reason 3: Confusing "Spin" with Scientifically Valid Research

For vendors who are eager for health care providers to embrace their products or services, statistically valid research is nothing more than an impediment to overcome on the road to successful sales. Research is replaced by rhetoric, and "spin" becomes substituted for science.

Sometimes this spin comes in the form of "evidence-based" guidelines that purport to be grounded in impeccable science but may be more marketing than medical science. Several thousand such guidelines have been published by a plethora of organizations.[13]

Dr. Otis Brawley, chief medical officer of the American Cancer Society, observed that "this is precisely what happens when professional societies of doctors who perform expensive medical procedures issue 'evidence-based guidelines' that are anything but evidence-based guidelines. Instead, the purpose of many of these documents is to protect the specialties' financial stake in the system."[14] Such a sham denigrates the medical profession by promoting the ongoing use of inappropriate practices.

Danger, Will Robinson: A Case Study in Spin

We've always had a fascination with robots. Some of us are old enough to remember the iconic robot from *Lost in Space* that constantly warned the young Will Robinson of danger. In medicine, it turns out, not all robots are so helpful. Even so, one manufacturer, Intuitive Surgical, is pulling out all the stops to convince you otherwise.

The DaVinci surgical robot, first introduced by Intuitive Surgical in 1999, soon became a staple of the modern operating room. Demand for the equipment soared, according to an article appearing in the August 19, 2010, issue of the *New England Journal of Medicine*, stating that "robotic technology has been adopted rapidly over the past four years in both the United States and Europe. The number of robot-assisted procedures that are performed worldwide has nearly tripled since 2007, from 80,000 to 205,000. Between 2007 and 2009, the number of DaVinci systems, the leading robotic technology, that were installed in U.S. hospitals grew by approximately 75 percent from almost 800 to around 1,400."[15]

The exponential growth curve for surgical robots continues. In 2012, the number of robotically assisted surgeries grew to 367,000—representing more than 25 percent growth over the prior year's volume, according to Intuitive Surgical.[16]

Far from inexpensive, these machines represent major capital investments by hospitals strapped for cash. The cost may exceed $2 million per robot. But the costs do not stop with the acquisition of the machine. There are also maintenance contracts that can approach $500,000 annually, as well as surgical supplies costing $1,500 per case. All in all, it makes for one expensive tool! Yet most hospital CEOs will tell you that it's a small price to pay for a hot technology in great demand by patients and surgeons.

It may be "hot," but what's most striking about this rate of adoption is the lack of evidence showing proof of the superiority of the treatment. In a research study published in the *New England Journal of Medicine*, authors Gabriel Barbash and Sherry Glied determined that robot-assisted surgery generally raised the cost of the procedure by 13 percent when the amortized cost of the equipment was included. They also determined that there did not appear to be any gains in efficacy or reduction of adverse effects for the most commonly performed robotic procedures such as prostatectomies. Rather, there was simply a reduction in postoperative recovery time.[17]

Dr. Brawley seconds this contention, stating that "almost all studies comparing robotic surgery to conventional surgery haven't demonstrated significant advantages."[18]

Such was the case with my friend, Tom, who needed a radical prostatectomy due to a particularly aggressive cancer. Tom was more fixated on finding a hospital armed with a robot than locating the best urologist to perform his procedure. He did not want to hear a word about what the data demonstrated. Instead, he repeated phrases that could have been lifted straight from marketing information . . . glowing promises of great outcomes and a speedy recovery.

When a man is facing the prospect of incontinence or impotency, two relatively common side effects of radical prostatectomy, it is understandable when they seek out any solution promising a brighter future. Unfortunately, despite its convincing propaganda, there isn't enough evidence to support the use of robotics in place of human hands.

The lack of improved efficacy associated with robotic surgery applies to more than just prostatectomies. According to a study of more than 260,000 hysterectomy patients published in the *Journal of the American Medical Association*, patients fared no better under the robot than under the knife. There was an important difference, however, in these two groups: "The median hospital cost for robot-assisted surgery was $8,868, compared with $6,679 for a laparoscopic hysterectomy. The study found that although patients who got robotic hysterectomies were less likely than laparoscopic patients to be hospitalized for more than two days, there was no significant difference between the two groups on other measures, such as complications and blood transfusion rates."[19]

Robotic surgery is not merely more expensive; some experts allege that it is also more dangerous. There are two reasons for the added danger. First, the bulky robots purportedly impeded emergency CPR during surgery, according to some anesthesiologists.[20] For a patient whose heart has ceased beating, the robot may have stood in the way of his resuscitation.

Another reason for the increased danger associated with robotic surgery is allegedly due to the inadequate training of surgeons. It's generally accepted that "surgeons must perform 150 to 250 procedures to become adept in their use."[21] Yet a recent article appearing in the *New York Times* berated Intuitive Surgical with well-supported accusations that its salespeople used inappropriate tactics to have poorly qualified surgeons performing procedures. "In an e-mail dated May 31, 2011," the *Times* wrote, "a Western regional sales manager for Intuitive noted that area surgeons had used robotic equipment only five times, although the company's goal was to see thirty-six robotic operations performed by the end of June. He urged sales staff to persuade surgeons to switch upcoming cases to robotic ones. 'Don't let proctoring or credentialing'—shorthand for supervised surgery and hospital certification—'get in our way,' the e-mail said."[22]

If the robot's higher costs (with no meaningful difference in clinical outcomes other than slightly reduced lengths of stay), coupled with its alleged risks, are insufficient to shake your confidence in this new modality, then also consider the number of unnecessary surgeries being attributed to the robot.

Massive marketing of the robot to physicians by Intuitive, coupled with marketing to consumers by hospitals hungry for some point of competitive advantage, may have contributed to "an increase of more than 60 percent in the number of hospital discharges for prostatectomy (including both robotic and traditional procedures) in the United States between 2005 and 2008. This increase occurred despite a decrease in the underlying incidence of prostate cancer and contemporaneously with a striking increase in the number of robot-assisted prostatectomies performed in the United States."[23]

How aggressively do hospitals market the robot? Dr. Makary, aided by one of his medical students, Linda Jin, examined hospital websites for marketing claims relative to their DaVinci Robot. The research demonstrated that "robotic surgery is being actively marketed on 41 percent of U.S. hospital websites, many of which make unsupported claims of robotic surgery's superiority."[24] Frustrated by the lack of meaningful evidence justifying the use of the robot, Makary further commented, "When I get a few beers into my colleagues who promote robotic surgery, they too will often admit that it's mainly a marketing hook to attract patients."[25]

Robotic surgery is but the tip of the proverbial iceberg when it comes to arguably inappropriate use of medical interventions.

Using Radiation to Pad the Pocketbook

When it comes to prostate cancer, the surgical robot must compete with two other, nonsurgical, treatment modalities that appear to offer comparable efficacy—IMRT and brachytherapy. Intensity-modulated radiotherapy (IMRT) is a highly focused form of radiation administered in a series of thirty-five to forty-five treatments. Brachytherapy involves the implanting of radioactive "seeds" within the prostate. Though there are differences in the potential side effects associated with each method of treatment, one of the greatest differences relates to cost—and who profits from it.

IMRT is costly. A U.S. Government Accountability Office (GAO) study released in the summer of 2013 stated that the cost of IMRT for men diagnosed with prostate cancer in 2005 was nearly double ($31,575) that of either a surgical prostatectomy (approximately $16,500) or brachytherapy ($17,076).[26]

Eyeing a cash bonanza, many urological groups across the nation invested in radiation-therapy centers capable of administering IMRT. These physicians profited handsomely by recommending IMRT to their patients over other alternatives—including surgery. Furthermore, these physicians were not required to disclose their vested financial interests to their patient.

Perhaps that's why the GAO discovered that "the number of and expenditures for Medicare prostate cancer–related IMRT services performed by self-referring groups grew rapidly from 2006 through 2010."[27] The number actually increased more than 450 percent from

80,000 IMRT procedures to 366,000, raising Medicare's tab for this procedure from $52 million to $190 million during the same period. The GAO further concluded that the overall growth in the use of IMRT for prostate cancer was "entirely due to an increase in the services performed by limited-specialty groups"—a.k.a. urologists. [28]

These are the same specialists who a number of years earlier made tremendous profits through the administration of androgen-deprivation therapy for prostate cancer. These monthly injections, given in physician offices, accounted for as much as 40 percent of the total revenue some urologists collected in a given year. [29] When Medicare slashed reimbursement on the drugs, their utilization by urologists dropped precipitously.

Let me be quite clear: There are no prohibitions against any of these activities. Furthermore, far from being an unproven therapy, IMRT is often the treatment of choice with prostate cancer patients. Therefore one could argue that the urologists were simply capitalizing on the financial benefits associated with providing selective modalities of care, as do numerous other specialists who also emphasize highly reimbursed procedures. In so doing they were ensuring the financial stability and success of their practice. Conversely, though playing by the rules of the game, such practices nonetheless raise profound issues regarding our health care system's tolerance for potential conflicts of interest.

Reason 4: Greed, the Nail in the Coffin of Medicine

When the size of the health care "pie" is $2.8 trillion and growing, plenty of people line up at the trough to be fed. That's why the most powerful reason for delivering unproven therapies to patients is plain and simple greed. These interventions, irrespective of their efficacy, efficiency, or safety, are guaranteed to generate money, and few people are invulnerable to the siren song of cash—including physicians.

Some of America's leading physicians have broken ranks by stating that greed is a plague upon the industry and a cancer within the profession of medicine. Though doctors are far from the only ones with dirty hands when it comes to putting profits ahead of patients, it is doctors on whom we rely to maintain the integrity of medicine. They are the self-anointed stewards of the industry and enjoy the benefits of such power and should act in a manner that justifies the public's trust. But when physicians are encumbered by conflicts of interests between the needs of the patient and the interests of the doctor, trouble is sure to arise.

Dr. Arnold Relman is among the most outspoken critics of this shift in the culture of medicine. In his powerful book *Second Opinion* he says that "physicians are supposed to be fiduciaries for their patients, so financial ties to the facilities and technology that they use for their patients create an obvious conflict of interest. These conflicts of interest now pervade the practice of medicine, and they inevitably increase medical expenditures because they encourage physicians to use the facilities, procedures, tests, drugs, and medical devices in which they have a financial interest, without sufficient consideration of cost and benefits or the availability of alternatives that may be less expensive and just as good or better."[30]

Relman isn't alone. In 2010, the Institute of Medicine stated clearly that "large numbers of physicians have pharmaceutical, hospital, and other financial relationships that consumers are unaware of but likely create influential fiduciary relationships in conflict with those of consumers."[31]

Dr. Makary, a physician on the front lines of medicine, said this assault on the traditional values of medicine has become a daily occurrence. "By my estimate," Makary calculates, "financial incentives lure the average doctor two to ten times a day, temptations that are not always ignored—particularly when treating patients with borderline indications, who comprise a large part of the patient population."[32]

Physicians become either active participants or pawns in the efforts of the medical-industrial complex to raise the nation's health care bill while further lining their pockets.

A GLUT OF TREATMENTS

One has to wonder whether the early adoption of controversial and unproven forms of treatment would have flourished without a strong profit motive. Before attempting to answer that question, let's examine an egregious example of money before good medicine—the use of bone-marrow transplant (BMT) procedures in the treatment of Stage IV breast cancer.

Stage IV breast cancer patients have a very high mortality rate due to the systemic progression of the disease. Though the cancer's advance may be slowed for varying periods of time (remissions), rarely is such advanced cancer cured. Unfortunately, metastatic breast cancer takes a heavy toll as measured in deaths each year.

Such high stakes have attracted the attention of researchers across the globe. In 1989, without any clear scientific rationale to support their actions, some doctors began experimentally treating metastatic breast cancer patients using BMT.

According to George Lundberg, MD, such procedures were "dangerous, debilitating, and expensive. Between 15 and 20 percent of the patients died from the drugs used in the procedure. Many others had permanent injuries, including heart damage and hearing loss. And the procedure cost upward of $200,000."[33]

Despite the lack of evidence supporting the procedure's efficacy, as well as its tremendously high costs and potentially catastrophic side effects, there was explosive growth in the use of the procedure over the next two decades. In fact, breast cancer patients militantly demanded that their insurers pay for it.

In communities where insurance coverage was not an option, "well-meaning people throughout the United States held community bake sales and charity raffles to raise money for a bone-marrow transplantation for a breast cancer patient in their midst. The friends and neighbors had no idea that they were helping some doctor get rich on an unproven procedure that harmed the patient."[34]

Over time, it was revealed that some of the data supporting the use of BMT for metastatic breast cancer had been falsified. Three of four studies showed no benefit. "The last study was the only one to suggest that there could be beneficial results from bone-marrow transplants, but the claim collapsed when outside researchers discovered that the South African data had been falsified."[35]

Few physicians can speak more authoritatively to this malfeasance than Otis Brawley, who stated that "the number of women who were unwittingly, unnecessarily—and, yes, fraudulently—harmed by this procedure is staggering. Between 1989 and 2001, at least twenty-three thousand women underwent the procedure outside clinical trials. Some estimates are much higher—thirty-five thousand to forty thousand."[36]

MATTERS OF THE HEART

Cancer patients aren't the only ones exposed to expensive and arguably unnecessary treatments. Heart-disease patients suffer a similar fate—facing risky, expensive procedures of indeterminate benefit.

Many of today's heart procedures are designed to relieve atherosclerosis—a narrowing of the arteries that channel blood to and from the heart. Some of the most common and lucrative procedures are intended to achieve "revascularization"—improved blood flow, presumably to ameliorate symptoms and reduce cardiac deaths. These procedures are often the economic lifeblood of a hospital. They are performed· on a routine basis, day in and day out, presumably whether needed or not.

Paul Chan is a world-renowned cardiovascular researcher based at the Mid America Heart Institute in Kansas City. In 2012, Chan et al. published a study in the *Journal of the American Medical Association* that examined whether physicians were appropriate in their usage of percutaneous coronary angioplasties—a procedure in which a catheter containing an inflatable balloon is inserted into a blocked artery. Once inflated, the balloon compresses the occlusion, allowing free blood-flow. Oftentimes, a stent is left in place to aid in keeping the vessel open.

Chan's research showed a profound lack of evidence supporting the seemingly indiscriminate use of this treatment in patients. "Of the roughly two hundred thousand heart angioplasty procedures done in the United States each year for patients without heart-attack symptoms," he wrote, "38 percent are done for uncertain indications, and 12 percent (or roughly twenty-four thousand) are done for 'inappropriate' indications."[37]

Chan's work, along with numerous other studies, have helped earn the United States the dubious distinction of having the "highest rates of coronary revascularization procedures, with more than double the rates of other countries," despite having "similar mortality rates from heart disease."[38]

Beyond utilization rates, researchers also investigate clinical outcomes associated with various cardiac procedures. One study, conducted by Yusuf et al., compared procedural outcomes for heart patients across six countries.[39] Two of the countries, Brazil and the United

States, performed the greatest numbers of revascularization procedures. As a result, patients in both countries benefited from a reduction
in one of the major symptoms of heart disease—refractory angina. But,
perhaps even more importantly, this study also showed no gain relative
to reductions in heart attacks or death from cardiovascular events. In
fact, the risk of stroke was elevated.[40]

The rewards for performing such procedures are high, and cardiologists are certainly not immune from the allure of procedurally generated revenue. Dr. Mark Midei, a cardiologist trained at the venerable
Johns Hopkins, was no exception.

Dr. Midei was one of the most prolific utilizers of angioplasty and
stents. As his reputation grew, so, too, did his volume of implantable
stents—quickly rising to twelve hundred stents in a single year. Such
huge volumes sometimes garner attention, as proved to be the case with
Dr. Midei.

In a story appearing in the *New York Times*, author Gardiner Harris
quotes an investigatory senatorial report stating that Dr. Midei "may
have implanted 585 stents [that] were medically unnecessary" over a
two-year period—for which Medicare was billed $6.6 million in
charges.[41] It appears that the hospital with which he was aligned may
have been complicit by allegedly providing Midei with economic incentives tied to his patient volumes.[42]

Before angioplasty was so commonplace, open-heart surgery was the
preferred method for revascularization. Among some physicians, for
certain patients, it is still the option of choice. The popularity of open-
heart surgery can be seen in our comparative usage rates. The U.S. rate
of open-heart surgery (coronary-artery bypass) was almost double the
OECD median (184 percent greater) in 2010. Only Germany exceeded
our rate.[43]

Such data causes one to pause, once again, and question the appropriateness of the frequency of these procedures. Do U.S. doctors know
something that is oblique to physicians in other advanced nations?

Not according to Nortin Hadler, MD, a professor of medicine at the
University of North Carolina. In his book *The Last Well Person*, Dr.
Hadler went so far as to denounce revascularization procedures as a
form of malpractice by questioning the very science supporting it.
"Based upon compelling and robust science," he wrote, "interventional
cardiology and cardiovascular surgery for ischemic disease stemming

from atherosclerosis fit the criteria for Type II Medical Malpractice," which he describes as "doing something to patients very well that was not needed in the first place."[44]

Different surgeries have vastly different levels of recovery and risk. When it comes to coronary-artery bypass grafting (CABG), Hadler asserts that "the surgical community does little to forewarn us of the demonstrated downside of these procedures." He goes on to delineate the downside:

> The anguish of the cardiac catheterizations required before surgery, the challenges of healing and recovery, the 2 to 8 percent who die on the table or in the postoperative period, the 50 percent who suffer emotional distress, mainly depression, in the first six months, the 40 percent who have memory loss at a year, and the alarming number (depending on their level of activity before the CABG) who never return to the workforce or describe themselves again as well and enjoying life. For some, dementia is the only clinically important result of having their coronary-artery anatomy successfully rearranged. For none is the likelihood of survival improved.[45]

Hadler's position may be extreme, but so, too, may be the level of frequency with which we crack open people's chests in the hope of ameliorating the effects of heart disease.

A PAIN IN THE NECK

Other frequently performed but controversial forms of surgery are those procedures intended to alleviate common back or spine problems. I learned this firsthand a decade ago when a bulging disc in my neck—a condition that is often referred to as a *herniated disc*—brought me to my knees in pain while on a trip to Washington, D.C. After a sleepless night in my hotel room, I took a cab to the emergency room at Inova Health System. The ER physician ordered a shot of Demerol to relieve the pain, combined with Valium to stop the associated muscles spasms. My sense of relief was immediate, though I'm still mystified as to how I made it safely back to the hotel so laden with drugs (the hospital staff made sure I was safely ensconced in a cab and that the driver had clear instructions to return me to my hotel in one piece).

When I returned home, I paid a visit to a neurosurgeon at a local hospital. The surgeon took one look at my MRI and told me that I needed surgery. No ifs, ands, or buts, and I was to have it the next day. He went on to state that, because we were friends, he would be sure that the hospital would accommodate me.

It was about then that I remembered that this surgeon had been described to me as the hospital's golden goose (one of its top revenue generators). He achieved this distinction by virtue of the number of expensive procedures he performed. I thanked him for his time and promptly left his office.

My unremitting pain drove me to visit another neurosurgeon across town. This particular surgeon enjoyed an impeccable clinical reputation. Thanks to the intervention of a mutual friend, this well-respected doctor was able to work me in the next day. He pored over my MRI, meticulously examined my spine, and listened intently to my description of the pain and chain of events after the herniation. Then he looked me squarely in the eyes and said, "I would avoid surgery at all costs unless you absolutely cannot stand the pain."

He went on to explain that there was a reasonable chance of my condition resolving without intervention. My recommended treatment: some daily exercises coupled with over-the-counter anti-inflammatories/pain relievers, and a healthy dose of patience. That was thirteen years ago. Though the problem flares on occasion, the pain is neither sufficiently strong nor enduring to necessitate a return visit to the doctor.

This surgeon performed exactly as physicians should perform 100 percent of the time. He unflinchingly put my needs ahead of his gains. The result, in this case, was no surgery. As you can imagine, I never heard a word from the first neurosurgeon. I'm sure he found someone else to operate on.

Spine patients, as a group, may derive little benefit from surgery, whether necessary or not. Neurosurgeons, however, can derive tremendous financial benefit from performing such procedures. Not only do they collect sizable professional fees, but sometimes there is even an added kicker, as was the case with five neurosurgeons in Kentucky, detailed by Makary:

In 2009, that group preformed the third-highest number of spinal fusions in the country on Medicare patients. In addition to what Medicare paid them with tax dollars, the surgeons received $7 million directly from Medtronic, the company that makes the metal implants.

Were those procedures warranted? Who knows? But I can say with confidence that spinal fusions are in a controversial gray area. Conservative back surgeons maintain that degenerative-disc disease (the most commonly cited indication that spinal fusion is required) does not require surgery and can be treated just as effectively with physical therapy and pain medication.[46]

The problem does not lie solely with the efficacy of the surgery but equally with our expectations about the aches and pains that are part and parcel of the human condition: "It is normal to have degenerative changes of the musculoskeletal system. If you have a pristine spine at midlife, that is distinctly 'abnormal.'"[47]

But it is our very refusal to tolerate the discomfort of aging that has made spine surgery into another major profit center for many hospitals. And though it is highly lucrative, a myriad of clinical trials have shown it to be of dubious effectiveness in eliminating various forms of back and neck pain.

According to Dr. Hadler, "there are more than two hundred randomized controlled trials of treatments for axial pain, yet none of the various forms of poking, prodding, injecting, exercising, yanking, girding, needling, and the like can be shown to consistently and robustly offer any advantage over placebo effect."[48]

THE COMPLICATED CASE OF MASTECTOMIES

The discussion thus far could lead one to the erroneous conclusion that issues of medical treatment are black or white. So let's examine one that is more "gray." There's no better example than the use of mastectomies to treat Stage I breast cancer.

Unlike Stage IV breast cancer, a designation of Stage I indicates no systemic progression of the disease. It is also defined by limitations on the size of the tumor and other factors. The prognosis for the vast majority of women with this disease is quite good—often a cure.

For years, however, the treatment of choice for *any* stage of breast cancer was a mastectomy: "Surgeons performed disfiguring radical procedures called the Halsted mastectomies for more than seventy-five years because William Stewart Halsted said it was the right way to treat breast cancer."[49] Though the surgery was an injury to both their psyche and soma, for most women, it was far better than living in the shadow of cancer.

In the 1960s a small cadre of surgeons, including Oliver Cope, began to wonder whether this radical surgery was necessary to beat cancer. "Cope, a professor of surgery at the Massachusetts General Hospital, realized that the radical mastectomy had not discernibly improved the five-year survival of patients compared to historical controls."[50] So what type of surgery was truly indicated for women presenting with early-stage breast cancer?

The answer to such an important question could not hinge on intuition. "It took an iconoclast—Bernie Fisher, a surgeon at the University of Pittsburgh—to stage a randomized clinical trial that demonstrated that a conservative procedure followed by radiation was equivalent to radical mastectomy [for certain women]."[51]

Fisher's research team limited their study to women meeting the criteria for early-stage breast cancer. What they—and subsequent researchers—discovered was that the "radical mastectomy, rather than heroic, turned out to be mutilating."[52] Study after study would demonstrate that a vastly less-invasive procedure, the lumpectomy, when combined with postsurgical radiation, was equally effective in treating Stage I breast cancer for the vast majority of women.

Three decades later, however, mastectomies are still commonly performed for the treatment of Stage I breast cancer. Why would otherwise healthy women select a more difficult and disfiguring surgery over a procedure from which they can recover in a few weeks? Theories abound on this topic, but several hypotheses are worthy of mention.

Let's begin by looking at how breast cancer is positioned in the minds of the public. The American Cancer Society and Susan G. Komen for the Cure have done an excellent job of alerting women to the threat of breast cancer, as well as to its potential consequences. The medical community has taken up arms to battle it in the *war against cancer*. Therefore, when the enemy appears, it strikes incredible fear into any woman's heart. At such times, she is profoundly vulnerable.

The choices a newly diagnosed cancer patient makes may be greatly influenced by the level of unbiased information she receives from her physicians at this critical juncture. Even a gentle nudge in the direction of mastectomy over lumpectomy is usually all that's required for a patient to select this procedure. That nudge may come from her primary care physician, medical oncologist, radiation oncologist, surgeon, breast cancer navigator, or even a behind-the-fence neighbor who happens to be a breast cancer survivor.

There is ample evidence that physicians may be unknowingly complicit in steering the patient toward mastectomy. As will be discussed at length shortly, researchers at the Dartmouth Atlas project have shown tremendous unexplainable geographic variation in the level of mastectomies versus lumpectomies for Stage I breast cancer.[53]

Another factor influencing our patient may be the stories of famous celebrities who have gone public with information about their mastectomies. For some patients—such as Angelina Jolie—who harbor genes that predispose them to virulent forms of breast cancer, mastectomy or double mastectomy is a logical choice. The percentage of such women in the overall population, however, pales in comparison to the volume of mastectomies performed on "normal" women with early-stage cancers.

Mastectomies illustrate the power of comparative-effectiveness research—showing that women with early-stage breast cancer truly can choose between treatments with comparable efficacy. There is no right or wrong choice here . . . as long as the choice a woman makes comes from an informed perspective. Unfortunately, "our system's virtues have broken down to the point at which whether you get a minimally invasive versus large open operation depends on surgeon 'style' (with the patients unaware). Is this the freedom of the 'art' of medicine—or the chaos of subprime real estate before the crash?"[54]

Perhaps in the near future, the focus of Susan G. Komen for the Cure will move beyond heightening breast cancer awareness, a topic now indelibly etched into the consciousness of most Americans, and turn toward the issues of informed, collaborative decision making between cancer patients and their care providers.

WHEN CANCER IS NOT MALIGNANT

Sometimes women are thrown into a full-blown anxiety attack by a diagnosis that isn't even cancer—DCIS being a prime example. Though pathology textbooks have stated for decades that DCIS, or ductal carcinoma in situ, is not a true malignancy, it has somehow mutated in popular understanding into cancer. The American Cancer Society's chief medical officer, Otis Brawley, offered the observation that "sometime in the 1980s, a group of breast cancer advocates and advocacy organizations started referring to DCIS as *breast cancer*. Doctors and surgical oncologists started doing this, too. The pathologists never wavered, but because everyone else started calling it *cancer* over the past twenty-five years it's become cancer."[55]

Once given a diagnosis of cancer, patients are understandably eager to take action; and this includes far more than just DCIS patients. In July 2013, the National Cancer Institute published the recommendations of a working group examining the definition of *cancer*. The group concluded that not only should conditions such as DCIS be renamed to eliminate the word *cancer* but other relatively benign conditions, such as thyroid nodules, should also be clearly labeled as such to mitigate unnecessary, expensive, and painful interventions.

I recently underwent a carotid-artery ultrasound to rule out a potential serious circulatory problem. In the process, the technician spotted something suspicious in my thyroid gland. The radiologist confirmed that it was a nodule measuring approximately 1.5 centimeters and was of undefined origin. "There's a small chance it's cancer," I was told. "A needle biopsy would give us more information" followed.

Fortunately, my wife believes in watchful waiting. On the small chance that it is a cancer, it will likely grow very, very slowly and will be contained. The least invasive and relatively inexpensive option is to repeat the ultrasound after six to twelve months and observe any changes in the size of the lesion. That's what I'm opting for. I'll let you know how it turns out.

A LESS MALIGNANT BUT MORE UBIQUITOUS PROBLEM IN MEDICINE: OVERUTILIZATION OF TESTS

When we go to our physician for an annual physical or a minor illness, we give little thought to the boxes he or she checks as blood work is ordered. We are far more focused on that painful needle stick that we are about to endure. Yet research shows that "about 80 percent of lab tests now ordered are not needed by anyone other than laboratory directors, hospital administrators, and often physicians, and many are priced at scandalously high levels. These are scattershot tests encouraged by lab-ordering forms and by physicians accustomed to asking for any and all test results."[56]

The costs of these "scandalously" priced tests add up. According to journalist Steven Brill, writing in *Time* magazine, "about $70 billion will be spent in the U.S. on about seven billion lab tests in 2013. That's about $223 a person for sixteen tests per person. Cutting the ordering and overpricing could easily take $25 billion out of that bill."[57]

It's not just lab tests but diagnostic imaging as well. Once again, the United States outstrips every other developed nation relative to the number of such tests—performing one thousand MRIs and more than 250 CTs per one thousand population.[58] That's "more than twice the average in other OECD countries."[59]

A number of factors undoubtedly contribute to this staggering level of overutilization, including that (1) we've made ordering tests phenomenally easy for physicians—and it may be easier to order a complete panel than the handful of individual tests that will have utility for the patient; (2) comprehensive testing may help safeguard the wary physician from malpractice claims; (3) patients demand a testing modality, such as MRI, without any real appreciation of the clinical appropriateness of their demand; and (4) someone is profiting from the screening, either directly or indirectly.

The current poster child for unnecessary testing is the PSA test. The level of PSA, or prostate-specific antigen, can be measured with a simple blood test. PSA tends to rise when a patient develops prostate cancer. Therefore, elevated PSA levels have been viewed as a prognostic indicator for the potential presence of cancer. But the story is far more complicated. First we need to understand a bit about prostate cancer.

Virtually every man will develop prostate cancer if he lives long enough. However, very few men will die sooner as a result of the disease. Though there are virulent forms of it, it is generally more indolent in presentation and takes years, if not decades, to develop. As the chief medical officer of the American Cancer Society so succinctly put it, "despite concerted efforts, screening for prostate cancer has not been clearly proven to decrease men's chances of dying of prostate cancer."[60]

So why screen? Even the government has weighed in with an opinion on the "need" for screening:

> The U.S. Preventive Services Task Force recently released a draft recommendation on screening for prostate cancer, designed for primary care physicians and health systems, and has opened it for public comments until November 8, 2011. After completing a rigorous evidence review, the task force decided to recommend against screening for prostate-specific antigen (PSA), concluding that there is moderate or high certainty that the service has no net benefit or that the harms outweigh the benefits. This grade-D recommendation applies to healthy men of all ages, regardless of race or family history.
>
> The task force points out that no trial showed a decrease in overall mortality with the use of PSA-based screening through eleven years of follow-up and that all trials showed either a small or no benefit in prostate-cancer-specific mortality.[61]

These are not new findings. Hadler, writing in 2004, stated that "the futility of prostate screening is obvious from the results of several randomized controlled trials that have been published."[62] Unfortunately, no one seemed to be listening.

With reams of data stacked against PSA screening, why has its use been so prolific in the industry? The answer to this question may be hidden in the sequence of events that often follow a positive PSA test, probably beginning with a painful ultrasound-assisted biopsy of the prostate. If a cancerous lesion is detected, the patient then may face surgery or radiation to eradicate the disease.

Both treatments have significant side effects that can dramatically affect the patient's lifestyle but not necessarily his longevity: "The radical prostatectomy he may choose to undergo might provide a 50 percent decrease in the likelihood that he will die of prostate cancer. The procedure will, however, make little or no change in the timing of his death or the overall quality of his life. In 15 percent of patients, it is also likely to produce a major problem with erectile and urinary function."[63] Other physicians put the likelihood of impotence or incontinence far closer to 30-plus percent.

In all such cases, one thing remains constant: expensive treatment modalities will be used to rescue the patient from the uncertain fate of prostate cancer. As one author put it, "the PSA test underpins a prostate cancer industry, consisting of laboratories that do biopsies, manufacturers of surgical robots and radiation equipment, even suppliers of adult diapers."[64]

Dr. Brawley describes the intense marketing efforts of hospitals to capture potential prostate cancer through the "noble" act of free screenings:

> Call it "disease mongering" or call it the marketing of disease, but as I write this, a fleet of aquamarine, white, and blue mobile homes is bringing prostate cancer screening to a shopping-mall parking lot near you. These things are long, thirty-nine feet, plenty of room. Come aboard! The blood test is free, but the cascade of follow-up services will ring up considerable sales for treatments that leave guys impotent and incontinent. Treatment that *may* have a miniscule chance of saving them from cancer, but a much larger chance of treating a cancer that would never have harmed them, or may not even have been there in the first place.[65]

The American Urologic Association (AUA), rather than acting to protect the best interests of patients, appears to have been complicit in their fleecing by remaining silent on this issue. It was not until 2013 that the AUA finally "pulled back its strong support of prostate cancer screening, saying that the testing should be considered primarily by men aged fifty-five to sixty-nine."[66]

Fortunately there are professional medical societies that are trying to do the right thing. A case in point is the nine physician groups, under the leadership of the American Board of Internal Medicine Foundation, working to help minimize unnecessary testing and procedures. Each professional society has identified its top five tests or procedures most overutilized by the medical profession. These tests range from inappropriate indications for CT scans to the frequency with which colonoscopies are performed. A host of consumer-advocacy organizations is also working in partnership on the project.[67]

THE LESSONS LEARNED

There are three lessons that I hope you take away from this chapter. First is an admonition from Dr. George Lundberg: "The quality of the procedure is defined by its scientific efficacy. Difficult as this may be for patients, physicians, and hospitals to accept, we need to base medicine on science, not on hopes and dreams of cures and profit."[68]

The second lesson is that informed consent is an essential component of each and every treatment decision we make, yet truly informed consent may be a rarity based on a complex array of factors. Therefore, the burden of understanding our options, and what is ultimately in our best interest, falls disproportionately in our laps.

The third lesson is that physicians are divinely human and subject to the same foibles as you and I, including greed. Greed becomes a sin when it threatens to compromise informed-patient consent and the provision of appropriate care.

WHAT YOU CAN DO TO PROTECT YOUR HEALTH

Your best protection is to assume responsibility for your health by becoming the consummate consumer of health care services. That means you are prepared to ask questions until convinced that you possess the requisite information to make informed decisions about your care. On your journey, you may encounter physicians who, when questioned, appear outraged by your lack of blind faith and capitulation to their greater wisdom. When you meet such physicians, quickly part company.

Whether it is a "routine" blood test or open-heart surgery, you deserve to understand what is being done in the purported interest of your health, as well as whether these recommended tests or treatments are being driven by any conflicting interests. Finally, you must understand the potential outcomes from any intervention.

So let's begin with testing. First, get to know your physician's philosophy regarding preventive screenings, and the degree to which his or her practice guidelines line up with established standards. Since these guidelines are often age-specific, be sure you are interpreting things correctly. As we've seen with PSA testing, established standards are no guarantee of appropriateness, but they may be the best indicator that you, as a consumer, can rely on.

If your physician is recommending screenings that fall outside these guidelines, inquire as to why. You are not questioning his or her competency, merely why they are deviating from an established norm. Also remember that, just as there is overutilization, so, too, could you be a victim of underutilization. If your physician fails to recommend a routine screening that is age-appropriate, such as mammography, inquire as to why.

If a routine screening comes back positive, there's a new level of discernment that you need to engage in with your physician, including asking the following questions:

- How clinically significant are the findings?
- How conclusive (definitive) are the findings?
- What is the confidence level in the findings?
- What are the next steps to confirm, refute, or advance the findings?
- Should you be identifying potential specialists?

If your physician recommends additional testing, before consenting you should understand

- the nature of the test being recommended;
- the clinical indication or other justification for recommending it;
- what information will be gleaned from test results;
- how the test results might influence the recommended treatment options;
- what, if any, dangers or complications can arise from the test;
- other dangers, such as false positives, that will require further testing to rule out;
- how urgent the perceived need for the test is;
- what the cost/benefit of the test is; and
- how much discomfort or pain you will experience as a result of the test.

Let's consider one area of screening—methods for detecting the potential presence of breast cancer (men get it, too). Beyond self-examination or palpation by a physician, the most common screening modality is mammography. While useful in identifying some tumors, it has many limitations—including high rates of false positives, poor results when screening women with dense breast tissue, and the inability to identify certain types of tumors that can proliferate undetected within the breast. Even so, it has utility as a preliminary screening method for the general population.

Other diagnostic-imaging modalities for identifying potential breast tumors include tomosynthesis, breast MRI, and ultrasound. Each technology has its unique strengths and weaknesses that should be explained to you by the physician ordering the test. If a suspicious "spot" is found in your breast and confirmed by multiple imaging modalities, your physician will likely order a stereotactic breast biopsy. Assuming it is properly performed, and the lesion in question is actually sampled with the needle inserted into the breast, it should help provide a definitive diagnosis of your condition.

Listen astutely to your physician and ask for clarification or elaboration as needed when addressing these issues. If you must see a specialist, you can either defer to your physician's recommendation or take a more proactive role in finding the best doctor for your particular condition. We will address this process in far more detail later.

Now that you understand what is being recommended to confirm or deny the existence of a potential harmful condition, you may wish to do some research on your own. If so, it is essential that you seek out trustworthy resources, as noted in the prior chapter. By way of reminder, some basic guidelines may help you separate "the wheat from the chaff," though they cannot guarantee the validity of the information so derived:

- Though far from flawless, peer-reviewed articles can be an excellent source of the latest research findings relative to the efficacy of tests and interventions. Unfortunately, these articles are often written in a language that is virtually impenetrable to mere mortals.
- The good news is that the mainstream media often report on research findings that are truly significant or applicable to large

portions of the population, as was the case with PSA testing. The bad news is that the research findings may be reported in a manner that is technically correct but misleading to the public.

- A great many books are printed every year examining issues of proper and improper utilization of medical tests and interventions. These, too, can be a valuable resource once vetted based on the degree to which they are impeccably researched by the author.
- Another source of generally trustworthy information is governmental websites, such as those sponsored by the Centers for Disease Control, the National Institutes of Health, and the Centers for Medicare and Medicaid Services.
- Finally, one may wish to consider sites sponsored by not-for-profit organizations, though the tax-exempt status of these sponsors is no guarantee of the veracity of the information they provide—as was seen with the American Urological Association.

If it sounds like a lot of work, it is; but what better payoff is there than the protection and preservation of your health?

When testing leads to the recommendation for specific treatments, another round of discernment begins. Your quest for knowledge should include determining the following:

- Ascertain the physician's confidence level in the diagnosis, as well as your own. Trust your gut, and don't hesitate to indicate your desire for a second opinion. You may opt to either have an additional specialist recommended by your physician or seek one out yourself.
- Assuming the diagnosis is correct, what are the options for treatment, and what is being recommended?
- What are the relative strengths and weaknesses of each approach?
- Are there unique aspects of your condition that make one option more appropriate than another?
- What type of specialists will need to be involved in your care based on the selection of a given option?
- Are there specialists in your area who possess the clinical skills required to effect a good outcome? Do they perform these procedures with appropriate frequency to maintain their clinical edge?

- How urgent is the treatment, and why?
- How costly is the treatment (relative to value gained)?
- Does the physician whom you have selected to perform the treatment have any economic interest in your chosen treatment that may encumber his or her objectivity?
- How arduous and lengthy will the recovery be after treatment?
- What are the common side effects of such treatment?
- What additional risks are associated with the treatment?
- What happens if you choose to do nothing?

It's easy to describe the methodical process required to make data-driven decisions for your care. What is profoundly difficult is working through such decisions at a time of crisis. If you've received a disheartening diagnosis, such as cancer, you may already be battling anxiety, elevated blood pressure, and more than a twinge of existential despair. So lean on loved ones to support you as you struggle to make the best decisions possible.

However, be careful to not rely on loved ones as a source of objective data. Friends and family can reliably report on the quality of personal interactions or experiences they have had with various providers, but they are far less reliable as expert witnesses relative to clinical capabilities or the clinical appropriateness of various tests and treatments. The exception may be the surgical nurse who has worked for twenty years at one major hospital, knows the good, the bad, and the ugly about every surgeon on staff, and just happens to be your neighbor.

An essential lesson that we will expand on in chapter 5 is that, though a recommended intervention may be absolutely appropriate for your condition, your personal outcome may vary dramatically based on who is performing the intervention at a given facility. It becomes vitally important, as we shall see, to understand which specialists practicing at which hospitals have the greatest experience and demonstrate the best outcomes relative to this treatment option. As we've already seen, even something as simple as the number of procedures a physician has performed can dramatically affect the procedure's outcome.

MYTH 4
"WHERE ONE CHOOSES TO RECEIVE CARE WILL HAVE NO BEARING ON THEIR TREATMENT OPTIONS, OUTCOMES, OR COST"

In the 1970s, Jackie Townley was a rough-and-tumble little boy growing up in Stowe, Vermont—a town known to many as the outdoor recreational capital of the state. It was a perfect place for a little boy who loved the cold bluster of a wintery day to grow up. He spent many an afternoon sledding with his friends or chasing a hockey puck across the frozen expanse of a neighbor's pond.

But Jackie increasingly missed the opportunity to play outside due to an almost chronic sore throat. After repeated bouts with tonsillitis, his pediatrician recommended a tonsillectomy. "No big deal," thought his parents, Karen and Tom, who had watched innumerable compatriots of Jackie undergo the procedure. A few weeks later, Jackie had his tonsils removed and was, once again, brimming with energy.

Ten miles away in Waterbury, Jenny Dobson, who loved making snowmen with her dad, was suffering from recurrent bouts of tonsillitis. Unlike her neighbor to the north, Jenny's pediatrician did not recommend surgery but, rather, elected to manage her condition with medication.

Though Jackie and Jenny are based on a composite of patients residing in these two adjacent communities, they illustrate the variations in care observed by a maverick researcher named Jack Wennberg, who lived between Stowe and Waterbury. He began to have a hunch. In his gut, Wennberg believed that he was witnessing inexplicable and substantial variation in the medical practices (practice patterns) of these otherwise similar communities. If medicine was predicated purely on scientific evidence, it should not matter whether one lived in Waterbury or Stowe, or for that matter, Peoria or the Poconos. One would expect a level of consistency in treatment.[1]

Wennberg knew he needed impeccable data to support such a controversial allegation. Aided by fellow researcher Alan Gittelsohn, Wennberg analyzed the rates of tonsillectomies in Waterbury and Stowe. In the process, he discovered that children in Stowe were three and half times more likely to have their tonsils surgically removed by the age of fifteen than their counterparts in Waterbury.[2] Though it would take many years for the full impact of Wennberg's hunch and resulting research to be felt, it would eventually rock the world of health care.

Wennberg and his colleagues were on the path to demonstrating that "in health care, as in real estate, it all boils down to location, location, location."[3]

A MAVERICK RESEARCHER SHINES A LIGHT ON VARIATIONS IN CARE

Fueled by his early discovery and in quest of an explanation for why there was such variance in the use of a common surgical procedure, Wennberg, aided by Gittelsohn, embarked on a systematic analysis of health care utilization across the state of Vermont. The two researchers divided the state into thirteen geographic regions and methodically examined how patients were treated in each.

The results, at the time, were groundbreaking: Wennberg "found that patients admitted with the same disease, the same symptoms, the same insurance, and the same resources available to help them were treated very differently at the two locations. It was an amazing disclosure."[4]

As they had hypothesized based on their casual observations of tonsillectomies, Wennberg and Gittelsohn proved that there was wide variation in the frequency of nine of the most common surgical procedures. The greatest variance was seen in tonsillectomy, "which varied from a low of 13 to a high of 151 cases per 10,000 persons."[5]

There was also substantial variation in the amount of money spent on health care. Wennberg and Gittelsohn showed a more than 100 percent variation in the level of spending per capita for hospital services in 1969.[6]

Despite these stunning revelations, when it came time to publish their data Wennberg and Gittelsohn were met with rejection by all the traditional medical journals. Undaunted and eager to share their findings with the scientific community, the two men finally sent their article to *Science*, a well-respected journal. The editors at *Science* recognized that Wennberg and Gittelsohn had a powerful and well-researched story to tell.

The article appeared in the December 1973 issue of *Science* and was greeted with little fanfare despite, or perhaps because of, its provocative message. When seeking to explain the more than 1100 percent variation in the frequency of tonsillectomies, the authors concluded, "There are no data available that would allow us to relate these variations to the prevalence of tonsillitis, but it appears that the variations are more likely to be associated with difference in beliefs among physicians concerning the indication for, and efficacy of, the procedure."[7]

But wait a minute . . . how could variation be caused by the *beliefs* of physicians? Is not medicine supposed to be empirical rather than philosophical?

Another provocative finding reported in the article was that "the supply of general surgeons is positively related to the surgery rate at all levels of surgical complexity and for nearly all types of individual procedures."[8]

Still there was no outcry.

BUILDING AN EVEN STRONGER CASE BY GATHERING MORE EVIDENCE

Undaunted by the lack of fanfare, Wennberg and Gittelsohn continued their work—expanding the geographic scope of research to include other northeastern areas. "In one Maine city, for instance, they discovered that hysterectomies were so frequent that if they continued at the same pace, '70 percent of the women there will have had the operation by the time they reach the age of 75.'"[9]

Each new discovery catalyzed interest within the research community. Though the research effort was exceedingly slow to build, a team of astute researchers joined Wennberg over the ensuing two decades, analyzing variation in clinical utilization patterns on an enormously expanded scale. No longer was the northeast the sole purview of Wennberg's scrutiny. Now the entire United States was fair game.

In a March 4, 1993, issue of the *New England Journal of Medicine*, Wennberg et al. took on the topic of "Geographic Variation in Expenditures for Physicians' Services in the United States" by examining Medicare data for the 317 major cities and towns in the United States. They employed sophisticated methods for ensuring "apples-to-apples" comparisons across communities—adjusting for age, sex, and other factors.

The article concluded that not only was there a tremendous variation in the number of hospital admissions based on geography, but there was also an equally dramatic variation in the payment to physicians for caring for these hospital patients. "The admission rate per 1,000 beneficiaries (mean 304) ranged from 219 in Boise, Idaho, to 533 in Pascagoula, Mississippi," they found. "After adjustment for price and case mix, payments to physicians for inpatient care per admission (mean $1,180) ranged from $677 in Vancouver, Washington, to $1,580 in Miami."[10] As with his earliest work, Wennberg's research raised as many questions as it answered.

At about this same time, Wennberg began work on what was to become the Dartmouth Atlas. The Atlas was originally intended to help power the proposed Clinton health care reform efforts. When the Clinton-era reforms failed, Wennberg scrambled to find a new use for his powerful data. He decided to make the information available to numerous public audiences in an effort to drive change.

As a result, it was first published in 1996. In 2000, the Dartmouth Atlas was published on the Web, making "a strong nationwide case for what had been observed only in regions before: the kind of health care you receive depends on where you live rather than what is wrong with you."[11]

CARRY ON, MY WAYWARD SON

Today the work begun by Jack Wennberg and Alan Gittelsohn, once considered rogue, is viewed as providing an invaluable window into the dramatic manner in which health care varies by setting. Best of all, this data is not squirreled away behind impenetrable firewalls but is available to you on the Web.

Take a look for yourself by visiting the Atlas online.[12] With a little practice, you will be able to unlock the power of the database. In the interim, there are preformatted reports that may be of great interest.

Let's take a brief look at some of the findings from the 2012 *Dartmouth Atlas Report Highlighting the New England Region*:

- "If you have heart disease and live in Winsted, Connecticut, you are half as likely to undergo balloon angioplasty than if you live in Marlborough, Massachusetts, and more than twice as likely to undergo back surgery than if you live in Manchester, New Hampshire. If you have osteoarthritis of the knee and live in Calais, Maine, you are twice as likely to have your knee replaced than if you live in Providence, Rhode Island."[13]
- "Among the largest twenty communities in New England, we found fivefold variation in PSA testing for prostate cancer and nearly threefold variation in radical prostatectomy rates."[14]
- "The greatest variation was seen in mastectomy for breast cancer. Among the twenty largest communities, rates of mastectomy varied more than fivefold, ranging from a low of 0.3 per one thousand female Medicare beneficiaries in Springfield, Massachusetts, to 1.5 per one thousand in Hyannis, Massachusetts."[15]
- "Similar variation can be seen in the usage of [coronary artery bypass graft] to treat stable angina. There is a more than fivefold variation from low to high across the U.S."[16]

These types of variations hold up when we expand our focus from the New England region to the nation. A good example can be seen in the treatment of prostate issues. Many men in their fifties and sixties experience prostate-related problems, with symptoms such as urinary retention, a sense of urgency relative to urination, and even blockage. The underlying culprit responsible for this discomfort is usually BPH, or benign prostate hypertrophy. Though not particularly dangerous, BPH is not always easy to live with on a daily basis, as I've learned.

The treatments for BPH span a broad gamut—from "watchful waiting" to radical prostatectomy. "Of all the treatment options, surgery offers the best chance for improved symptoms, along with the highest risk of complications and side effects. The most common type of surgery is called a transurethral resection of the prostate (TURP)."[17]

There was a sixteenfold variation in the manner in which BPH is treated even within a highly contained hospital-referral region encompassing Seattle. Whether it is watchful waiting, pharmacotherapy, or the scalpel, based on the stunning level of variation, the "choice" appears to be more driven by who is delivering the care and where than by the condition of a man's prostate.

At times, men suffer the symptoms of BPH due to a somewhat less-innocuous condition, prostate cancer. Similar variations were seen in the rates of radical prostatectomy used to treat prostate cancer. There was a tenfold variation nationally.[18]

DIVIDING VARIATION IN TWO

In an interview published on the Dartmouth Atlas website, Wennberg stated that there are two major types of variation in health care in the United States—one being a function of supply and the other being caused by style. "One is extremely related to supply of resources—how many doctors there are, how many beds there are, how much ancillary services are available," said Wennberg. "This quantity of capacity drastically affects the intensity with which chronically ill people are treated from one part of the country to another. And this is the source of the huge differences in overall Medicare spending, the fact that spending in Miami is nearly twice that . . . of Minnesota or Portland, Oregon."[19]

The other major finding or focus is on surgical procedure, variations in the rates of knee replacements, hip replacements, gallbladder surgery, heart surgery, carotid-artery surgery, you name it, where the surgical variation is essentially one side of the equation. On the other side of the equation is the alternative way of treating the same condition. What we see here, then, are situations where the practice patterns reflect underlying differences in opinion about whether one treatment should be used or another treatment should be used.[20]

The implication of Wennberg's first finding seems to be that health care, once again, circumvents market dynamics. In highly competitive markets where the supply of products or services is in abundance, the price generally declines. In health care, however, providers drive up the level of utilization to match supply.

Wennberg's second finding is easily illustrated by example. Let's take a look at a hypothetical patient, Jennifer Taylor.

Jennifer Taylor lives with her family in a quiet community just outside Grand Forks, North Dakota. Her husband, Robert, is a retired Air Force officer who was last stationed in Minot. The couple's two grown children, Sarah and Susan, live within an hour's drive, allowing Jennifer and Robert to spend plenty of time with their grandchildren.

Both Jennifer and Robert are extraordinarily diligent about taking care of themselves. They want to be around for a long time and watch their grandchildren grow and thrive. Jennifer never misses her annual mammogram—particularly now that she was approaching sixty.

In 2012, a routine screening identified what appeared to be an early-stage tumor in her right breast. An MRI corroborated the finding, and a subsequent needle biopsy provided the undisputed proof. Terrified by the word cancer, Jennifer urgently sought the advice of her physicians.

She was told that her tumor was approximately one centimeter across and that there was no evidence that it had spread to her lymph system—though this would not be known for certain until her lymph nodes had been biopsied. In the absence of any evidence that it had spread beyond the local site, Jennifer appeared to have an early stage or Stage I cancer—a disease that is highly curable. Also in her favor was the lack of familial history of cancer. So there was little concern that Jennifer would possess the rare genetic mutations that trigger aggressive forms of cancer.

Her medical oncologist recommended a mastectomy and referred her to his preferred surgeon, who agreed that a mastectomy was the treatment of choice. Though she was provided with the option of having a lumpectomy, Jennifer said, "It was quite clear what these two men thought was in my best interest."

As we saw in the previous chapter, in cases such as Jennifer's, the scientific evidence supports both procedures equally. The lumpectomy followed by a short course of radiation appears to be as effective in curing cancer (eliminating the primary occurrence and preventing subsequent recurrence) as mastectomy—and is obviously far less invasive, disfiguring, and expensive. Furthermore, it has a far shorter recovery time. Had she been provided with this information, Jennifer states that she would have made a very different decision. She would have been spared significant surgery—including the cosmetic reconstruction of her right breast.

What Jennifer—and virtually all patients—fail to understand is the degree to which geography determines destiny when it comes to their health care. Had Jennifer lived in San Francisco, odds are that her physicians would have recommended a lumpectomy. In fact, the variation in mastectomy rates nationally ranged from a low of 0.3 per one thousand in San Francisco to a high of 2.3 per one thousand in Grand Forks, North Dakota—a nearly 800 percent variation![21]

As noted by Wennberg, this type of variation is frequently seen for procedures where the evidence of efficacy is either equivocal or completely absent, as is the case with back surgery. Brownlee et al. tried to explain rationally the sevenfold variation they observed in back-surgery rates across the country. The conclusion they came to was that "differences in clinicians' personal beliefs and opinions contribute to the variation in surgical rates in different geographic locations. For example, there is considerable disagreement among surgeons about the need for back surgery, its effectiveness, and even the best way to diagnose the cause of the back pain. With no consensus about how to diagnose and treat back pain, the rate of back surgery varies widely from place to place."[22]

The work of Wennberg, Brownlee, and others adds up to one powerful conclusion: "Much of what we do has no scientific evidence behind it. So by that token, most variation is what we call 'unwarranted'—it can't be explained by those factors."[23]

THE COST OF VARIATION

The key to efficiency is minimization of variation in process. When processes are tightly standardized, quality goes up and costs go down. In health care, that means better, safer, and cheaper care.

What does variation in health care cost the nation? Based on work done by Wennberg and his colleagues in 2002, the Dartmouth group estimated that regional variations in care amounted to approximately 30 percent of our national health care bill or $750 billion in 2009.[24]

Numerous researchers at organizations ranging from the McKinsey Global Institute to the Commonwealth Foundation have reached similar conclusions regarding the excessive costs brought about by variation. Most of this research is powered by the Dartmouth Atlas.

Thirty percent of a $2.8 trillion national health care tab is a mind-numbing number. If you have trouble swallowing it, here are a few facts regarding variation in cost that may help lend credence to this bold assertion:

- "Medicare spends 2.5 times as much on its Miami enrollees as it docs on those in Minneapolis—for no good reason and with apparently worse outcomes."[25]
- "Such variation is also unfair because workers and Medicare beneficiaries in low-cost, more-efficient regions subsidize the care of those in high-cost regions."[26]
- "In a 2003 study, another Dartmouth team, led by the internist Elliott Fisher, examined the treatment received by a million elderly Americans diagnosed with colon or rectal cancer, a hip fracture, or a heart attack. They found that patients in higher-spending regions received 60 percent more care than elsewhere. Yet they did no better than other patients, whether this was measured in terms of survival, their ability to function, or satisfaction with the care they received. If anything, they seemed to do worse."[27]
- "To make matters worse, Fisher found that patients in high-cost areas were actually less likely to receive low-cost preventive services. . . . They got more of the stuff that cost more but not more of what they needed."[28]

I want to be certain that you retain one critical point from this data—a point that goes beyond cataloging the extreme levels of variation in care: The level of money spent on Medicare patients, coupled with the intensity of medical services they received, were far from the determinants of how a patient fared medically. In fact, *the evidence seems to suggest that more care is worse care* in terms of patient outcomes.

PATIENTS PAY THE HIGHEST COST

The price a patient pays cannot be measured solely by what comes out of their pocketbook. There are equally important variables in the equation, including whether they truly understood their options, they adequately expressed their preferences, and had their wishes honored by their physician—which was the issue that arose in Jennifer Taylor's situation. "The patient's preference for the kind of care he or she wants is especially important when facing a test, surgery, or other treatment that is 'elective,'" say Brownlee et al. "When a treatment is elective, it means there is more than one way to treat the patient's illness or condition, each possible treatment involves different trade-offs, and individual patients will view those trade-offs differently. Sometimes, doing nothing at first—'watchful waiting'—may be a completely reasonable option."[29]

When patients are given the objective, scientifically valid information that they need to make smart decisions about what is in their best interests, they are then involved in shared decision making with their providers. Unfortunately, "all too often patients facing the possibility of elective surgery"—surgery where there is more than one accepted standard for treatment—"are not given an opportunity to understand their options fully. Many patients are not even aware that the decision about elective surgery is actually a choice and that it should generally be theirs to make. Instead, they routinely delegate such important, even life-altering decisions to their clinicians in the belief that 'the doctor knows best.' The result is that patients often do not get the treatment that they would prefer."[30]

STANDING ON THE SHOULDERS OF GIANTS: GAWANDE BUILDS ON WENNBERG'S WORK

Atul Gawande, professor of Surgery at Harvard Medical School and professor of Health Policy and Management at the Harvard School of Public Health, writes prolifically about the status of American medicine. And through much of his work, the influence of Jack Wennberg is clear.

The June 1, 2009, issue of the *New Yorker* featured an article by Gawande, "The Cost Conundrum" (reprinted from the *Annals of Medicine*), in which the author traveled to one of the highest-cost health care markets in the country—McAllen, Texas—where, "in 2006, Medicare spent fifteen thousand dollars per enrollee . . . almost twice the national average."[31]

Gawande was on a quest to discover the source of the aberrantly high costs. He knew from reviewing the data that these aberrations were not due to a "sicker" population. In fact, "public-health statistics show that cardiovascular-disease rates in the county are actually lower than average, probably because its smoking rates are quite low. Rates of asthma, HIV, infant mortality, cancer, and injury are lower, too [than those of nearby areas with much lower costs]."[32]

Wanting to be certain of his facts, Gawande enlisted not only Dartmouth researcher Jonathan Skinner to carefully analyze Medicare data but two independent companies as well. These researchers made some fascinating discoveries—particularly when comparing health care in McAllen to care delivered in neighboring El Paso:

> Between 2001 and 2005, critically ill Medicare patients received almost 50 percent more specialist visits in McAllen than in El Paso and were two-thirds more likely to see ten or more specialists in a six-month period. In 2005 and 2006, patients in McAllen received 20 percent more abdominal ultrasounds, 30 percent more bone-density studies, 60 percent more stress tests with echocardiography, 200 percent more nerve-conduction studies to diagnose carpal-tunnel syndrome, and 550 percent more urine-flow studies to diagnose prostate troubles. They received one-fifth to two-thirds more gallbladder operations, knee replacements, breast biopsies, and bladder scopes. They also received two to three times as many pacemakers, implantable defibrillators, cardiac-bypass operations, carotid endarterecto-

mies, and coronary-artery stents. The primary cause of McAllen's extreme costs was, very simply, the across-the-board overuse of medicine.[33]

On-site interviews with providers in McAllen not only corroborated these findings but helped illuminate what had gone so terribly wrong with this town's health care. Providers had capitulated to the forces of greed and put profits ahead of patients: "So here, along the banks of the Rio Grande, in the Square Dance Capital of the World, a medical community came to treat patients the way subprime-mortgage lenders treated home buyers: as profit centers."[34]

Fortunately, not all towns and cities operate like McAllen—not yet, anyway. There are notable exceptions, such as Grand Junction, Colorado, "one of the lowest-cost markets in the country" and "a community of 120,000 that nonetheless has achieved some of Medicare's highest quality-of-care scores."[35] Rochester, Minnesota, home to the Mayo Clinic, also has remarkably affordable and clinically superb care.

> This doesn't mean you have to live near a world-class medical center to have the best shot at surviving a heart attack. What it does mean, surprisingly, is that where you live is an indicator of just how often you will see your doctor or a specialist, how many MRIs and other diagnostic tests you will have, and when your doctor will tell you that you need an operation.[36]

Gawande concludes by stating that "when you look across the spectrum from Grand Junction to McAllen—and the almost threefold difference in the costs of care—you come to realize that we are witnessing a battle for the soul of American medicine."[37] For him, the jury is still out, though the ethos of American medicine is leaning precipitously in the wrong direction. For others, the battle has already been lost.

WHAT YOU CAN DO TO PROTECT YOUR HEALTH

You may not be willing to pull up stakes and move from one locale to another to receive more appropriate care, but, at the very least, you should know how your location stacks up relative to the rest of the nation. You can then delve even deeper into how your hospital and doctor compare. But more on that later.

The Dartmouth Atlas can be accessed by anyone with a computer. Don't be intimidated by charts, graphs, or words you don't understand. Give yourself time, and it will begin to make a great deal of sense. Begin by familiarizing yourself with all the navigation features available on the site . . . and then begin to experiment. Be sure to look at many of the preformatted reports that have been generated in which researchers have done all the heavy lifting for you—not only analyzing the data but also drawing the appropriate inferences and conclusions.

If you live in an area where there is significant deviation from the norm in important areas of health care utilization, you need to be on your guard. Consider it a caution sign that there may be curves in the road ahead. The same principle would, of course, hold true if looking at comparative hospital data within your hometown.

If Jennifer Taylor had realized that her hometown had the highest rate of mastectomies for Stage I breast cancer in the nation, perhaps she would have sought out a second opinion from a leading cancer provider in another area. Her decision ultimately may have been the same, but there would have been comfort in knowing that it was reached in an objective, shared manner with her physician.

MYTH 5
"ALL PHYSICIANS ARE CREATED EQUAL"

A diagnosis of cancer is devastating. What's equally devastating is going through months of difficult treatment believing that you have a deadly disease, only to find out later that your physician erred in diagnosis. Yet that's exactly what happened to fifty-four-year-old mother of four Herlinda Garcia. [1]

After discovering a lump in her breast, Garcia went to see Dr. Ahmad Qadri, a board-certified medical oncologist/hematologist who had been in practice for more than twenty years. Upon his recommendation, Garcia had a lumpectomy whereby the tumor was excised and examined.

As the weeks following her surgery passed with little news from her physician, Garcia's anxiety began to build. Then came the call: Dr. Qadri informed Garcia that she was suffering from Stage IV breast cancer. [2] *Cure would not be an option, and her only hope of prolonged survival would be through a debilitating regimen of chemotherapy.*

In her mind, Garcia had no choice but to trust Qadri's diagnosis and treatment recommendation. She would spend the next seven months getting her affairs in order while enduring eight rounds of chemotherapy. [3] *Just as the harsh chemo agents took a toll on her physical body, the prospect of a dramatically shortened life damaged her psyche. By the time treatment ended, Garcia was sufficiently anxious and depressed that she sought medical help for these symptoms.*

As part of her medical evaluation for anxiety, a physician at Citizen's Medical Center in Victoria, Texas, evaluated the progression of her cancer. There was only one problem—he couldn't find it.[4] Suspicious that something was terribly amiss, the physician sent Garcia to the world-renowned MD Anderson Cancer Center in Houston "where she was tested, her original records reviewed, and it was revealed that she never had cancer and never needed chemotherapy."[5]

A flood of emotions swept over Garcia. She was tremendously relieved to have the death sentence lifted yet simultaneously angry at the tumultuous journey she had been made to endure by a physician's incompetence. Dr. Qadri had misread the pathology report on Garcia's tumor.[6] It was benign . . . not cancerous.

Had Garcia's case been presented in a tumor board, which is standard procedure in many cancer centers, the findings, prognosis, and treatment plan would have been critiqued by an interdisciplinary group of physicians. It's hard to imagine that the error would not have been detected almost instantly. But Garcia was not so lucky. No one was looking over the shoulder of Dr. Qadri. Nor did Garcia think to question him or seek a second opinion. . . . She put her full faith and trust behind her doctor and prayed that somehow she would make it through the ordeal.

Dr. Ahmad Qadri died in March 2013. Herlinda Garcia was awarded $367,500 for the anguish she had endured . . . an award to be paid by the estate of Dr. Qadri.[7]

Medical errors are commonplace. Sometimes they are an almost inevitable consequence of the complexities of medicine intersecting with the fallibility of human beings. Other times, however, they are due to incompetence, impairment, or other preventable factors that put patients in harm's way.

I've watched as a surgeon, who was too drunk to operate, left a bar and headed straight to the OR in response to a call. I've watched the calamitous impact of a fire breaking out in an OR suite and injuring the patient. And I've been privy to the egregious errors reviewed in medical executive committees where the discussions would remain safely ensconced in a veil of secrecy.

REPLACING BLIND TRUST WITH RESPECTFUL DISCERNMENT

The trust we place in our physicians is part of the very foundation of American medicine. Unlike other professions, in medicine trust does not have to be earned by its practitioners. Rather, it is bestowed on every doctor upon earning their MD.

Implicit trust in our doctors is like a curtsy or bow in the presence of royalty. Based on what we know today, this blind trust is not only unwarranted, it is dangerous. What is called for in its place is respectful discernment on the part of the patient and the expectation of collaboration when determining what care is required. Unfortunately, that's easier said than done.

Why do physicians enjoy a uniquely privileged role in our society—a role in which their life-and-death decisions are beyond public scrutiny? For three primary reasons—beginning with a need that is inherent in humankind: our need to believe in the power of a privileged caste to shield us from life's suffering while keeping death at bay. In primitive societies, it was the role of the shaman. In contemporary societies, that power has been bestowed on physicians.

Second, American medicine has solidified its cultural foothold by taking an already horrifically complex field and further ladening it with a unique brand of jargon—demanding a skilled translator. Medical jargon serves to reinforce our belief in the discipline's scientific rigor while simultaneously rendering its clinical observations and treatment recommendations impenetrable to mere mortals. A sweaty patient is *diaphoretic*. A patient with no appetite is *anorectic*. And a dead patient, similar to a parking meter, has *expired*. The implied argument is that surely individuals scholarly enough to discern meaning in these arcane terms are due respect.

Finally, much of the power enjoyed by our doctors is a testament to the extraordinary efforts of the American Medical Association (AMA). Over more than a century, the AMA has worked relentlessly to convince us of the impeccability of its scientific practitioners while trampling any competing schools of thought or methods of healing. Homeopathy, osteopathy, chiropractic, Chinese medicine, and other forms of "alternative healing" have struggled to establish legitimacy under the reign of the AMA.

If we put aside the issues of catering to our human frailty, masking the simple in the arcane, and lobbying to ensure the power of their profession, the question still remains, Are physicians due our respect?

For the vast majority of doctors, the unequivocal answer is yes. It is respect that is hard earned through years of personal sacrifice during medical training and practice. You can often identify these physicians by their humility. For some, humility is born from staring death and disease in the face while realizing the limitations of their art to intervene. For others, it is rooted in compassion and respect for their patients.

For the minority, however, the answer is no, for they have broken their sacred covenant to "bear a fiduciary trust in regard to their patients' health care needs . . . physicians agree to place their patients' health before any other outcome or goal and swear an oath to act as their patients' health care advocates."[8] In medicine, a few bad apples can indeed spoil the lot. As we shall see, medicine has done an abysmal job of culling out the bad.

Thank goodness for the small cadre of physicians concerned enough with the profession's negative trajectory to break ranks and speak out in impassioned condemnation. Among them is George Lundberg, who served as editor of the *Journal of the American Medical Association* (*JAMA*) for seventeen years and had this to say about the profession: "During my lifetime in medicine, I have witnessed a disastrous severance of trust, one that has led to runaway costs, constrained access, skewed coverage, and diminished quality. We cannot fix the American health care delivery system until we restore trust in medicine. Proper disclosure, assurance of access to scientifically proven therapies and preventive services, and complete patient and family participation are among the critical changes that must be made to mend our broken system."[9]

These are the reasons behind my call for *respectful discernment*. Respectful discernment means we go into every encounter with the medical profession with our eyes wide open. We know that not all doctors are created equal. And we are willing to take on the job of trying to find only the good apples.

SEEKING OUT THE GOOD APPLES

In your health care journey, nothing exceeds the importance of finding the right physicians for you or your family—beginning with the all-important primary care doctor. He or she will be your tour guide any time you embark on an adventure in the confusing realm of health care. The decisions you and your physician reach collaboratively will, at critical moments, touch your life in a profound way. So before you begin this search, you need to establish both the criteria that will optimize your chances of success and a process for applying those criteria to prospective physicians.

The information you are seeking can be divided into two categories. The first contains the basics—Does the physician accept your insurance plan? Are his or her hours convenient and accessible? Is he or she accepting new patients? This information can be quickly gleaned via a telephone conversation with the office staff.

Our second category contains more vital information and can only be gleaned through a rock solid due-diligence process that combines Internet searches, speaking with friends or family, and, most important-ly, interviewing your potential doctor. Why go to all the trouble? Because this is one of the most important decisions you will make.

So what exactly are you looking to discover? That depends on which characteristics are most important to you in a physician. If you are simply seeking a warm body with an MD, then the first category of information may suffice. If, however, you are more discerning and want a lifelong partner who will help you make astute decisions about your health, then roll up your sleeves and get ready to go to work. You want the kind of doctor that journalist David Bornstein described in the *New York Times*. "Great doctors," Bornstein opined, "don't just diagnose diseases, prescribe medications and treat patients; they bring the full spectrum of their human capabilities to the compassionate care of others."[10]

How do you identify a "great" doctor? There are ten criteria I believe you should consider when evaluating a physician. Before we get started, though, there is one very important caveat: It will be impossible to evaluate anyone across all the criteria due to the complexity of the task and the dearth of comparative information. Simply remember that each bit of information you gather adds important grist to the decision-making mill as you seek to identify the best physician for you.

No. 1: Education

Your physician has made a tremendous investment in his or her education. With few exceptions, they have completed four years of postgraduate study, followed by a residency in their chosen specialty (including family practice or internal medical medicine). Residencies range from three to eight years in duration. A family-practice residency requires three years, whereas a plastic-surgery residency requires approximately five years. Some physicians will then further subspecialize by completing one or more years in fellowship training.

Over the past century, America's medical schools have worked arduously to standardize their curricula. Of the 141 accredited medical schools in the United States, all are members of the Association of American Medical Colleges, a not-for-profit association that seeks to elevate the standard of training across all educational facilities. Even so, there is still variation in training—particularly once a physician enters residency. This variation may account for a portion of the geographic variation documented in the Dartmouth Atlas.

Arguably, there is also a vast difference in the quality and rigor of education provided by different medical schools. Though the barriers to entry are high across the board, admission criteria nonetheless vary dramatically. Most of the top medical schools are aligned with prestigious universities, whose brands carry equal cachet—such as Harvard, Duke, Stanford, Johns Hopkins, or Penn.

U.S. News & World Report ranks the nation's medical schools annually. For a fee, they will also provide a report showing two key criteria for admission: (1) the average MCAT scores (a standardized test that all applicants to medical school must take) and (2) average undergraduate grade-point averages. Top-ranked schools, such as Stanford, may accept as few as 3 percent of their applicants. The average undergraduate GPA for students admitted to Stanford or other comparable schools, such as Johns Hopkins, runs close to 3.8 on a 4.0 scale. MCAT scores are also exceedingly high at these schools.[11]

State schools, by comparison, have slightly more lax standards. For example, in the latest data reported by *U.S. News & World Report*, the

University of Texas Health Science Center at San Antonio, which ranked sixty-eighth, accepted 14.2 percent of applicants.[12] Students' average MCAT scores run approximately 20 percent lower than at Stanford, and the average undergraduate GPA is 3.57. Similar results can be seen across a plethora of other schools. Mind you, it is no easy feat to matriculate to such schools, but the criteria for admission, nonetheless, are less demanding than those found at the most academically elite medical schools.[13]

It's more than just class rank or MCAT scores that determines where students matriculate. Some of the best and brightest students cannot afford the cost of tuition at the academically elite institutions, nor do they wish to be saddled with debt as they graduate from medical school. Full-time tuition at Stanford runs more than $47,000 per year. Harvard approaches $50,000. The University of Texas is a "paltry" $14,500 for in-state students. Remember that great physicians emerge from each university. Even so, there is a difference in the academic milieus across the 141 medical schools.

One secret you will probably never unlock is how your physician performed in medical school. As the old joke goes, What do you call someone who finished at the bottom of their class in medical school? "Doctor." There is one indicator for excellent academic performance— membership in AOA. Each year, a small cadre of physicians who performed exceptionally well academically is invited to join an honorary society known as Alpha Omega Alpha (AOA). The society's website states that "the top 25 percent of a medical-school class is eligible for nomination to the society, and up to 16 percent may be elected based on leadership, character, community service, and professionalism. Members may also be elected by chapters after demonstrating scholarly achievement and professional contributions and values during their careers in medicine. Distinguished professionals may also be elected to honorary membership."[14] Just as Phi Beta Kappa connotes an important level of achievement, so, too, does AOA.

Residency programs show similar variance in their exclusivity, though formal rankings are harder to come by. Two measures of such rankings are (1) the *U.S. News & World Report* rankings of teaching hospitals by department and (2) rankings based on the level of National Institutes of Health (NIH) research funding received by departments across the majority of medical schools. One Internet resource, ResidentPhysician, purports to provide rankings across seventeen medical departments among 123 academic medical centers.[15] It should be noted, however, that the data listed may not be current.

Where your physician trained does make a difference. How much of a difference is impossible to quantify. What is easily measured, however, is the depth of your physician's training. It is essential that you understand the level of generalized knowledge or specialized knowledge that your physician brings to the exam room via his or her formal education.

Since there are no official rules on holding oneself out to be a "specialist," experts abound in medicine. A general surgeon, for example, who lacks formal fellowship training, may nonetheless proclaim that he or she is a breast surgeon simply by virtue of operating on such cases. An ENT may perform facial plastic-surgery procedures after only a short mentorship by a colleague. And a neurosurgeon may become an "expert" in deep-brain stimulation through a weekend course.

These physicians may be highly skilled and produce good outcomes, but there are factors not in their favor—beginning with the lack of formal, disciplined training, which also correlates with the number of cases performed in tandem with more experienced physicians before "flying solo." Says physician Marty Makary, "After I graduated medical school and got my license based on a 70 percent-or-higher passing score on my board exam, I was literally licensed to do anything in medicine— perform brain surgery, prescribe chemotherapy, remove varicose veins, or do electric-shock therapy for psychiatric disorders. I can legally do anything. In fact, some varicose-vein-removal centers in the United States are run by former ob-gyn doctors and others by psychiatrists; they were doctors looking to do something different and took a weekend course to learn how to do it."[16]

You probably don't want to be the third or fourth procedure a physician performs in their entire practice. Rather, you want to be their three- or four-hundredth such case performed over the past few years. Furthermore, you want to know that your doctor has received impeccable training.

There's nothing wrong with asking physicians about their education and level of training. Just bear in mind that it's just one data point . . . and there are nine more to consider!

No. 2: Certifications

Certifications provide an important way to differentiate among physicians. They do not ensure clinical excellence, compassion, or a moral compass, but they are a signpost . . . your second data point.

The most common and meaningful certifications are board eligibility and board certification. These require a physician to meet clearly defined criteria, as well as passing examinations held by the governing organizations over each specialty. Today many hospital medical staffs require board certification or board eligibility before granting privileges to practice at a hospital. There are excellent physicians without board certification and poor physicians with it. Therefore, it is simply a data point.

Case in point is a female physician in the Midwest. She labels herself a "breast surgeon." Her formal training was in general surgery, and she is neither board certified nor fellowship trained in breast surgery. Even so, most of her colleagues agree that her outcomes are excellent. Furthermore, she is well liked by her patients, who view her as very warm and empathic, traits not always found among surgeons. Would I recommend her to a family member? Yes, because I believe that she has proven herself consistently over time despite her lack of formal credentials.

Physicians may include other credentials in their marketing materials or business cards, including membership to specialized societies. In general, these designations say little more than that the physician or surgeon is a dues paying member of the organization.

No. 3: Knowledge

Because medicine is a rapidly evolving field, a physician's education is a lifelong endeavor. That's why there are requirements for continuing education in order to maintain licensure. Some physicians view continuing education as drudgery, while others are learners by disposition and want to have confidence that they are honoring their fiduciary obligation to the patient by staying current with medical knowledge.

A physician's knowledge can be measured by its breadth and depth. Your family practitioner or internist must possess robust knowledge about a broad array of medical topics, since they coordinate the totality of your care. Conversely, if you are seeing a subspecialist, you want them to possess a great depth of knowledge across a narrow range of topics.

Your physicians must be absolutely current on the latest findings and recommended treatment options related to your condition but not on unrelated medical matters. An epileptologist may, for example, know a great deal about cutting-edge methods for controlling seizures but would be a poor advisor on how to manage your recurrent back pain.

How your physicians acquire knowledge is also important, because it affects the reliability of that knowledge. Does she read peer-reviewed journal articles with a discerning eye? Does he attend medical conferences based on the quality of the presenters or based on the appeal of the conference locale? Does he search out trustworthy information or opinions when he has reached the limits of his knowledge? Does she understand the limits of her knowledge?

Unfortunately, physicians' ability to self-assess relative to the constraints of their knowledge may be limited. A meta-analysis of 725 articles on physician self-assessment published in *JAMA* in 2006 concluded that, "while suboptimal in quality, the preponderance of evidence suggests that physicians have a limited ability to accurately self-assess."[17]

You may never be able to assess your physician's knowledge, but you can make some assessment of style and inclination toward lifetime learning. One way to gain insight is to ask about the criteria on which your physician is making a recommendation. If he can cite current peer-reviewed research studies supporting his recommended interventions, then you can enjoy an added dose of confidence.

No. 4: Clinical Skill

If knowledge is difficult to assess, clinical skill is nearly impossible for the layperson to measure. For every clinical specialty, a unique set of skills is required. The pivotally important skill to an internist is deducing a patient's condition through a structured interview process, whereas one might argue that a surgeon's pivotal skill is the dexterity and adroitness with which she performs a procedure.

All specialties require strong cognitive skills—beginning with memory through deductive reasoning. Interventional skills require familiarity with techniques unique to the specialty and the knowledge and physical dexterity to execute these techniques with remarkable precision. Though we cannot easily measure relative skill, we can show tremendous variance across groups of physicians, as was demonstrated in a study of 10 radiologists who were each given the same set of 150 mammograms.

The physicians were not given any information about the patients' diagnoses or prognoses. They were simply asked to review the images and draw conclusions about what they observed. "For the mammograms from women who turned out to have cancer, the radiologists got the correct diagnosis between 74 percent and 96 percent of the time. For the mammograms from women who did not have the disease, cancer was highly suspected between 11 percent and 65 percent of the time."[18]

Though it's comforting that most cancerous lesions were identified, it is disconcerting that there were also a huge number of false positives—where no disease was present but the radiologists indicated it was *suspected*. The problem with a high rate of false positives is that they generate additional testing, unnecessary anxiety, and even unwarranted procedures.

Though there are undoubtedly innate variances in skill levels among physicians, studies have consistently demonstrated that physicians' skills are generally honed through experience. "A recent landmark research study published in the *New England Journal of Medicine* solidified what most doctors and nurses already knew," notes Dr. Marty Makary. "Using national data, a leading health services research group from the University of Michigan found that surgical death rates are directly related to a surgeon's experience with that particular operation. . . . Indeed, 'practice makes perfect' is a golden rule for medical procedures."[19] The study showed that, in the case of pancreas surgery, a surgeon who performed more than four such operations per year had a death rate of 4.6 percent compared to surgeons who performed fewer than two operations per year and had a death rate of 14.7 percent.[20]

There are dissenting opinions regarding the validity of volume as a predictor of quality. Charles Inlander, a prolific and outspoken consumer health care advocate, is impassioned about this point. According to Inlander, research conducted by the Pennsylvania Cost Containment Council clearly demonstrates that there are plenty of high-volume, low-quality providers out there. Therefore, he cautions, the notion that volume is directly related to quality is merely propaganda perpetuated by the industry.[21]

In Inlander's view, practice does not make perfect—particularly if one keeps repeating mistakes rather than refining technique. Perhaps a better way of looking at it is that volume is the ante a physician must pay to simply be in the game. For the physician to win your confidence, they have to demonstrate far more. If they're a proceduralist, that may include an ability to demonstrate minimal postoperative infection rates, few unscheduled returns to surgery within thirty days postoperatively, and positive outcomes relative to their peers.

If you ignore clinical skill altogether, you may run a big risk, as colorfully described by Otis Brawley, MD. "If you are rich, white, and insured, you face another deadly menace," says Brawley, "a socially prominent physician who is just plain bad. As a patient, you would see his social prominence—he might even belong to your country club—but you would have no way to see his inadequacy as a physician."[22] Dr. Makary describes this quintessentially bad doctor as "Dr. Hodad," an acronym for *hands of death and destruction*.

No. 5: Motivation

Physicians are as human as you or I. Trust me, I'm married to one. The truth is that I was drawn to my wife by the depth of her calling to heal people. Though she earns a good living, she lives a humble life. Much of her energy is devoted to her patients. She has reached into her own pocket on many occasions to help cover the cost of a prescription for a patient who had to decide between buying food or the medicine they needed to survive. Her motivation is tightly intertwined with her faith and her commitment to be a dutiful servant.

Though she's exceptional, she's not the exception. Many physicians bring a wonderful spirit of altruism to their practices. If you are fortunate, you have such a physician. If not, you may have a physician motivated by greed, pride, or other less noble virtues. It's not difficult to spot these physicians.

I was meeting with a specialist a number of years ago. It was a Monday—a busy day in his office. An elaborate board of lights alerted him to the status of each patient being seen that day. As a new light clicked on, in a classic Pavlovian response, he abruptly stopped the conversation and looked up. Realizing that Agnes, in the next room, was ready to be seen, he turned to me and said "Watch this! I'll be in and out in less than two minutes."

When he returned ninety seconds later, I asked "How do you do that?" He replied with a smile, "I do it all day long."

I hoped that Agnes had very few concerns or questions to discuss with her doctor that morning. Since this gentleman also took care of my aging mother, I shuddered to think of her waiting patiently to see him, only to then have a tornado-like experience as he blew in and out of the exam room with a fury.

Was he motivated by providing exemplary patient care or perhaps by how many patients he could churn in a given day? One needs neither be a saint nor sacrifice success to be a great physician, but one must be motivated by the right virtues.

You won't discern your physician's motivation on a website or by reading their marketing literature, which may position them next to Mother Teresa in terms of selfless altruism. Rather, you'll know it through the cues you receive every time you interact with them.

No. 6: Character Strengths and Virtues

Values are a close cousin to motivation. If motivation is what impels us, values are arguably the building blocks of our character.

Martin Seligman, past president of the American Psychological Association, and his late colleague Chris Peterson, a beloved professor at the University of Michigan, created one of the defining notions of positive psychology—that each of us possesses a unique constellation of character strengths and virtues that govern how we face the world. The team did not stop with a mere catalogue, however: Seligman and Peterson developed the Values in Action inventory (VIA) to identify the hierarchical importance of these twenty-four core strengths to anyone interested in taking a simple test.

Chances are you will not be successful in asking your physician to answer the three hundred questions that constitute the VIA inventory. However, you can become familiar enough with some of the VIA strengths to help determine which among them are most important to you when selecting a physician. Your own observations of your physician in action (PIA) may give you a sense of the degree to which your physician exemplifies these virtues.

When it comes to physicians, I would argue that one strength reigns supreme above all others in importance: *wisdom or perspective*. Seligman and Peterson suggest that, while the concept *wisdom* is seemingly easy to understand, it is far more difficult to define.[23] Kramer wrote in 2000 that wisdom "involves exceptional breadth and depth of knowledge about the conditions of life and human affairs and reflective judgment about the application of this knowledge."[24]

In our culture, wisdom is often equated with age, but don't be misled by whether your physician possesses gray hair. It is not the best indicator of wisdom. The thoughtful manner in which they collaborate with you to determine your care is a far more reliable indicator.

We had a young emergency medicine physician on staff at one of my hospitals. His extraordinarily youthful appearance earned him the nickname "Doogie Howser." More than once I had to counsel an anxious patient that Dr. de Leon was exceptionally well trained and accomplished. Once treated, his patients were universally impressed with his skills and manner.

Since collaboration on critical decisions is essential, you may wish to seek out a physician who is *open-minded*. "The open-minded thinker engages this style when confronted with an appropriately complex judgment in which evidence for and against a belief must be examined and weighed."[25] Due to the lack of comparative scientific evidence, much of medicine falls into this category. Therefore, you want someone who is not dogmatic but rather balanced in the manner they weigh evidence.

Based on the importance placed on education, it's only fitting that we would identify *love of learning* as an essential strength in a physician. "People who possess the general trait of love of learning are positively motivated to acquire new skills or knowledge or to build on existing skills and knowledge."[26]

So far, these values should be nonnegotiable. There are, however, values that may be more prized within a given context or specialty. *Bravery*, for instance, may be far less essential in the daily practice of family medicine than in cardiac surgery—where the surgeon may literally be holding your beating heart in their hands. Bravery is not simply about bravado in battle; rather, "bravery is the ability to do what needs to be done despite fear."[27]

I always applaud my wife's bravery when she has to give cancer patients bad news. Often she inherits patients who, though diagnosed by one or more prior physicians, are still completely in the dark as to their true condition. My wife has shared innumerable stories of patients whose bodies are ravaged by cancer, yet the word *cancer* has never been used by any of the patient's prior physicians. These are tough, sometimes gut-wrenching conversations, but they are essential if the physician and patient are to arrive at shared decisions regarding treatment.

For many patients, *kindness* is less a mandate than a wonderful touch of grace when evident in their physician. Peterson and Seligman define kindness as "the pervasive tendency to be nice to other people—to be compassionate and concerned about their welfare, to do favors for them, to perform good deeds, and to take care of them."[28] For me, kindness is an invaluable ingredient in the art of healing.

Two additional virtues are worthy of examination: *hope* and *spirituality*. Hope is often associated with optimism. And though most human beings want to remain hopeful in the face of adversity, I want my physician to be pessimistic—to be bedeviled with enough doubt to be thinking and rethinking whether he or she has rendered the proper diagnosis and prescribed the optimal treatment. Therefore, hope, while an essential virtue for all patients, is not on my PIA list.

Neither is *spirituality*, though it may be pivotally important to someone who is devout. Many patients receive tremendous comfort from doctors with whom they share similar spiritual and religious beliefs. Some physician practices have used their religiosity as the primary method for differentiating their practice. I'm fine with this proclamation of faith except for those cases of conscious hypocrisy that I've witnessed where clinics proclaim their religious identity but then behave in a manner antithetical to religious tenets.

Peterson and Seligman's book is eight hundred pages in length. I have done it a great injustice by so casually commandeering some of their concepts. I would strongly encourage you to take the VIA and see how true it rings for you. That will help you determine whether considering these values in action are meaningful when choosing a physician. The best way to become familiar with the VIA is by taking it.[29]

No. 7: Attention

Can your physician focus sufficiently on your needs to be effective? Will he or she take the requisite time to be an ombudsman for your care—whether advocating on your behalf with an insurance company or collaborating on a consult? Will you promptly receive the results of testing? And when you are acutely ill, will you get the immediate attention your condition demands?

There are many factors influencing the answers to these questions—beginning with the demands placed on a physician by virtue of their patient load. Also at play is their motivation, intrinsic ability to focus, stamina, and fatigue. A lack of attention can be annoying, disheartening, and even deadly. It's always disheartening to hear my wife describe cases in which a physician has failed to follow up on a positive diagnostic indicator for cancer, allowing the invading tumor to grow unchecked. By the time she sees the patient, the disease may be incurable. She can slow its progression, but the window for cure shut during the months in which it was ignored by the patient's primary care physician.

It would be easy to conclude that such inattention is purely the result of being a "bad" doctor, but it's far from that simple. There are numerous reasons why patients don't get the attention they need:

1. Health care is highly fragmented across specialties, treatment modalities, and sites of care. It is extraordinarily difficult for any physician to keep track of every intervention. It is difficult even to ensure that they have the complete history on their patients due to the multiplicity of sites often involved in diagnostic testing and treatment and the lack of a centralized repository for patients' histories and clinical data.
2. Many physicians operate under productivity quotas in which they are expected to see a certain number of patients in a given period. This "churn and burn" method of practicing medicine imposes a tremendous burden on physicians to remain attentive under adverse conditions.
3. Some physicians are less concerned about the appropriateness of care delivery and more interested in the level of reimbursement they can engender by taking shortcuts in care that result in profound inattention.

4. Finally, it's not all up to the doctor. Patients fail to do their part in appropriately reminding physicians of the need to discuss test results or next steps in care.

No. 8: Empathy

Empathy is a particular form of kindness that requires a physician to metaphorically place him- or herself in the patient's shoes and relate accordingly. In addition to being kind, empathy is validating—for it informs the patient of the physician's knowledge of and appreciation for their unique situation.

Empathy is a valuable gift. While essential in callings such as the clergy, it is nonessential but often highly valued when present in our physicians. Far too often, we hear the story of the dispassionate doctor who tells a patient that they have a terminal illness and then casually walks out of the exam room. No one with a shred of emotional intelligence would condone such behavior, but empathy is not a skill taught in medical school, nor is emotional intelligence measured by the MCAT.

No. 9: Impairment

Impairment caused by drugs, alcohol, or serious mental illness is never acceptable in a practicing physician. The problem lies in identifying the impaired physician, who may have well-honed skills for concealing their condition. Even when exposed, such issues are usually swept under the carpet by hospital and medical-staff leadership.

No. 10: Relative Costs

Our final method for differentiation among doctors is based on cost. Since doctors rarely if ever print a price list, this task can be formidable. Furthermore, we are generally one step removed from the physician's charges by virtue of our insurance coverage. We pay for the portion of the fee not covered by our insurance plan. If we paid straight out of our pockets without an intermediary, perhaps we'd be more cognizant of the relative value we receive from our doctors.

PHYSICIAN SELF-EVALUATIONS

As we have just acknowledged, it is extraordinarily difficult for a consumer to evaluate the clinical competency of a physician. If you don't believe me, doctors will be the first ones to tell you so! According to researchers James and Hammond, "Only another physician has the necessary knowledge and experience to judge whether a professional colleague adequately discharged his or her fiduciary trust to a particular patient."[30]

James goes on to state that doctors are so self-protective of their cultural status that "not only do physicians resist attempts of those outside the profession to inappropriately judge medical performance, they also insist on holding one another accountable for their performance within the profession of medicine."[31] Evidence suggests otherwise. Though they may "insist" on holding one another accountable, they do very little to honor it.

POLICING THEIR OWN RANKS TO PROTECT PATIENTS FROM DANGEROUS DOCTORS

If James's statement were true, the medical community bears a clear obligation to safeguard its patients' well-being by policing its ranks. Poor clinical performers, impaired physicians, and unethical practitioners should succumb to peer scrutiny or dramatically change their ways.

Theoretically, there are three levels at which such scrutiny should apply: (1) the peer-review committee of a hospital—which granted hospital-based privileges to the physician in the first place—(2) a state board of healing arts—responsible for ensuring the practice of safe and ethical medicine within the state—and (3) the ethics or disciplinary-action committees of national medical associations.

Unfortunately, a tremendous barrier stands in the way of effective reporting of physicians' malfeasance: the physicians' code of silence. Much like the mafia's *omertà*, it is an inviolate code of conduct inculcated into trainees early in their education. The message is simple: Don't attack your colleagues, or you might find yourself ostracized.

If you think I'm exaggerating, listen to what two nationally known physician-authors have to say on the topic, beginning with Dr. Makary:

Doctors and nurses know of docs who are reckless, but it takes moving a mountain to do something about it. Not reporting incompetence among peers is part of medical culture and has been for centuries. Medicine is poorly policed. Getting fired takes an action so egregious or offensive to hospital administration that I have only seen it happen twice among all the hospitals in which I've worked and trained.[32]

Dr. Brawley shares Dr. Makary's sentiment:

I know doctors who are just plain bad. Why do they continue to practice without impediment? The answer is simple: because no one is looking over their shoulders, no one files a disciplinary complaint, no tribunal of peers punishes them unless they do something spectacularly awful.[33]

PEER REVIEW: A PERFECT PATH TO BURYING PROBLEMS

When the level of suffering, injury, or unnecessary death inflicted by a colleague weighs too heavily on the conscience of some physicians, they can turn to peer review. The peer-review committee provides a venue for discussing and investigating allegations of inappropriate conduct by members of the medical staff. These allegations can run the gamut from violating standards of surgical appropriateness to boundary violations with patients.

In theory, peer review provides a fair and informed method for assessing the clinical or nonclinical behavior of a physician and the resulting potential for harm to patients. The proceedings are safeguarded against legal discovery—with the intent of promoting open, honest, and corrective dialogue.

Far from being effective, "such internal peer reviews are a little like the Russian parliament under Stalin," finds Makary. "No matter how much discussion there is, the results seems foreordained . . . any doctors who might raise probing questions are well aware that they can pay a heavy price for challenging their peers."[34] In those rare times when action is taken, the physician is often given the opportunity to simply resign their medical-staff privileges at a hospital or health system. By so doing, their misdeeds go unrecorded and they move across town to wreak havoc elsewhere.

I've seen physicians who fall asleep in the midst of complex surgeries, others who open up purportedly blocked arteries with multiple interventions—despite no discernible evidence of coronary disease. Some physicians knowingly inflict pain—either because they are sadistic or, more likely, because they don't want to waste time waiting for the effects of anesthetic agents to kick in.

The most outrageous case I know of involved a physician performing a circumcision on a two-year-old. The parents, waiting in a nearby room, heard their child screaming in pain. When later they asked the physician what had caused such a violent reaction in their child, he responded, "the injection of an anesthetic." In reality, he provided the child with no anesthetic—after all, it was a simple, quick procedure. In my mind there is a fitting punishment for such behavior on the part of the physician . . . and it is no mere slap on the wrist.

Finally, there are those who are blind drunk when operating. Such behavior is tolerated day in and day out in American medicine. To do otherwise would be to break the code of silence.

There are physicians who hold themselves to a higher code—one that demands owning responsibility for their actions. One such physician, Dr. Peter Elias, writing in the *New York Times'* Sunday Dialogue, offered this advice to his colleagues regarding medical error: "As a practicing family physician for thirty-six years, I have come to believe in the seven essential Rs of an apology: it should be Rapid (as in right away when the error is discovered), show true Remorse, Recognize explicitly the error, accept Responsibility, acknowledge the Repercussions for the patient, offer Restitution or repair, and close with a Repetition of the opening words: *I'm sorry.*"[35]

STATE MEDICAL BOARDS RECEIVE AN F FOR FAILING TO PROTECT US

A second "safeguard" against dangerous physicians should be state medical boards, which oversee licensure and disciplinary action. But they are not, according to Alan Levine, who provides oversight of the medical boards on behalf of the United States. Inspector General Levine indicates that many of these boards serve the vested interest of physicians to a far greater extent than they serve the public good.[36]

Though the accounts are anecdotal, I've heard many physicians suggest that these boards are partly populated by dangerous physicians. It's a case of the fox guarding the hen house. If there's bad news coming down the pike regarding a physician's practice, a position on the board will ensure that the physician will be first to hear it and attempt to squelch it.

In a recent review of state medical boards conducted by the consumer advocacy group Public Citizen, only two states were given an A rating. The vast majority received Fs. What was particularly disturbing was the variance seen among these boards. "The most recent three-year average state disciplinary rates (2009–2011) ranged from 1.33 serious actions per thousand physicians (South Carolina) to 6.79 actions per thousand physicians (Wyoming), a 5:1–fold difference in the rate of discipline between the best and worst state doctor disciplinary boards."[37]

Sidney Wolfe, MD, founder of Public Citizen, noted that there was no evidence to suggest that the rates of inappropriate behavior by physicians vary dramatically between states. Therefore, the variations observed by Public Citizen can only be attributable to the manner in which individual boards manage physician disciplinary issues. He goes on to state that "there is considerable evidence that most boards are underdisciplining physicians."[38]

Wolfe's research concludes that the average serious disciplinary rate, for any cause, is only 3.06 per one thousand . . . or 0.3 percent. Yet we know that there are a tremendous number of impaired physicians wreaking havoc on patients every day—physicians who obviously go either undetected or unpunished.

As Dr. Marty Makary points out in his book, *Unaccountable*, "There are also grossly impaired physicians [and] doctors with horrible skills, hazardous judgment, [and] ulterior motives or who suffer from substance abuse or other problems that make them dangerous. Society ought to be able to deal with this better, not sweep it all under the rug."[39]

Do such physicians represent the proverbial needle in the haystack and thus only affect an infinitesimally small portion of the population? Makary asks us to consider what it would look like if 2 percent of our doctors had a major impairment due to drugs, alcohol, or other causes. He then calculates that there would be twenty thousand impaired physicians in America treating up to ten million people per year.[40]

That's a lot of needles and haystacks.

If Makary's estimates sound absurdly high, consider the conclusions reached by researchers Eugene Boisaubin, MD, and Ruth Levine, MD, as published in the *American Journal of Medical Sciences*. "Approximately 15 percent of physicians," they find, "will be impaired at some point in their careers."[41] That's not to suggest that these physicians will, de facto, endanger their patients, but it certainly indicates a higher level of risk than might be suggested by the rate of disciplinary actions taken by state medical boards.

Caveat emptor to all patients: as Dr. Wolfe has demonstrated, "most states are not living up to their obligations to protect patients from doctors who are practicing medicine in a substandard manner."[42]

THE ABDICATION OF RESPONSIBILITY BY PROFESSIONAL SOCIETIES

The final level of protection from malevolent, incompetent, or impaired physicians resides in their professional associations—most prominently the AMA. The AMA's Code of Ethics states that "a physician shall deal honestly with patients and colleagues and strive to expose those physicians deficient in character or competence or who engage in fraud or deception."[43] The question becomes whether such standards are ever enforced. "After asking around," Makary found, "it became clear that the only time that a doctors' association would ever consider taking action against a doctor was if a state medical board had already done so."[44]

Professional societies exist not merely for the benefit of their members but to uphold the standards of the profession. Yet Otis Brawley, MD, questioned whether medicine even conforms to the definition of a profession. "A profession," he notes, "is a group of people who police themselves and put the welfare of their clients above their own. In many respects, people within medicine have forgotten what the word *profession* means."[45]

One can seek comfort in the belief that problematic physicians are few and far between, but the comfort will be short-lived. "An average American's combined exposure to quality failure from providers' underuse, overuse, and misuse of services is roughly 50 percent for preventive, acute, and chronic care services."[46]

IT'S TIME TO STEP UP TO THE PLATE: THE NEED FOR PHYSICIAN-DEFINED STANDARDS OF COMPETENCY AND REPORTING REQUIREMENTS

It is abundantly clear that there is a crying need to restore the fundamental trust between patients and physicians. A good starting point would be for the medical community to define criteria on which physicians' performances would be evaluated, as well as the degree to which such information would be transparent to the public. Right now, "there is no agreed-upon definition of competence that encompasses all important domains of professional medical practice."[47]

Doctors Epstein and Hundert, in an article published in *JAMA*, suggested a definition that, on the surface, appears quite cogent: "We propose that professional competence is the habitual and judicious use of communication, knowledge, technical skills, clinical reason, emotions, values, and reflection in daily practice for the benefit of the individual and community being served. Competence builds on a foundation of basic clinical skills, scientific knowledge, and moral development."[48]

The authors go on to discuss the importance of the following measures of competency:

- *Acquisition and use of knowledge.*
- *Integrative aspects of care.* "It is defined by the ability to manage ambiguous problems, tolerate uncertainty, and make decisions with limited information."[49]
- *Building therapeutic relationships.* "The quality of patient-physician relationship affects health and the recovery from illness, costs, and outcomes of chronic diseases by altering patients' understanding of their illnesses and reduction patient anxiety."[50]

- *Affective and moral dimensions.* "Moral and affective domains of practice may be evaluated more accurately by patients and peers than by licensing bodies or superiors."[51]

Epstein and Hundert also point out deficiencies in current methods for assessing competency: "Few assessments use measures such as participatory decision making that predict clinical outcomes in real practice. Few reliably assess clinical reasoning, system-based care, technology, and the patient-physician relationship."[52]

Finally, they point out, "Standardized test scores have been inversely correlated with empathy, responsibility, and tolerance."[53] Perhaps you should disregard what I said about MCAT scores.

In an interview in September 1997, I asked one of the physicians I revere the most how one finds a great doctor. Elisabeth Kübler-Ross, never shy of opinions, offered thoughts about why it is difficult to find a good doctor: "You have to be an A student. That eliminates 90 percent of the good people. Then you have to have lots of money—that eliminates the other few percent. That means it is pure coincidence if you get one good apple in the whole basket. Then you train them to cure, you don't train them how to be physicians."[54]

IS A BAD DOCTOR BETTER THAN NO DOCTOR? THE COMING SHORTAGE

Now that we know how arduous the process can be to find the right physician for you, let's add one more wrinkle. "The United States is in the middle of a primary health care workforce crisis that is expected to worsen precipitously in the next decade. The U.S. primary care workforce is undergoing a gradual but inexorable contraction that will seriously affect access to care."[55]

One of the primary drivers of this shortage is demographics. The baby boomers are aging—causing massive growth in the sixty-five-plus cohort of our population. Aging boomers will increase the demands on the health care system simply by virtue of their numbers and the requirements of managing their chronic conditions. Author Ken Dychtwald warned us of this impending phenomenon years before it happened in his book *Age Wave*.[56] Unfortunately, it appears that the right people were not listening.

As a result, we don't have enough doctors. The United States has approximately 22 percent fewer primary care physicians (PCPs) per thousand population than the OECD median.[57] "In the U.S., there are only about 1.2 primary care physicians per thousand people. In 2008, Spain had 3.6 practicing physicians per thousand people,[58] Canada had 2.3 per thousand,[59] Sweden had 3.6 per thousand,[60] and Germany had 3.5 per thousand."[61]

If we are to meet the growing demand for doctors, the Association of American Medical Colleges estimates that the United States will need ninety thousand more physicians by 2020, with forty-five thousand of them being primary care doctors. Medical schools are stepping up to the plate and increasing enrollment, but as early as 2016 there will not be adequate residency slots available to many of these graduate physicians.[62]

Another factor contributing to the shortage of PCPs is the differential in income between PCPs and other specialists: "If you look at the income gap, the average income of a PCP is only about 54 percent of what other specialties make. We clearly know that far more medical students choose to go into other disciplines rather than primary care. It's called the ROAD to success: Radiology, Orthopedics, Anesthesia, Dermatology. We know that over a lifetime, that gap in payment represents about $3 million in total income over one's career."[63]

Unless the situation changes dramatically, the shortage will be acute. Beggars can't be choosers, so pray that you can still use discernment when culling through a diminishing bushel of "apples."

THE WAL-MART OF HEALTH CARE

A sea change is occurring in the delivery of primary care, though many people have yet to feel its ripples. That change is coming in the form of retail clinics—a disruptive innovation that has arisen in response to the dearth of primary care specialists relative to growing demand, coupled with the costs incurred when utilizing a PCP's services.

Retail medicine takes the form of urgent-care clinics, usually housed in either a major retail pharmacy or big-box store and staffed by nurse practitioners. Though these health care workers lack the formal training of physicians, they are quite adept at dealing with a plethora of common problems ranging from upper-respiratory infections to minor wounds. Furthermore, they are guided by clear practice guidelines—ensuring a higher level of consistency in meeting standards of care.

Retail clinics are succeeding because they are cost efficient and more accessible and because they free up the PCP to act as a knowledge worker, not merely a technician. As Charles Inlander told me, "We are spending so much money to educate physicians, and then to have them come out and do throat swabs is a waste of money. We have given them very complex training, and we should use them to address the complex types of issues that people develop."[64]

How does mainstream medicine view retail clinics? In a recent interview, Doug Henley, MD, chief executive officer at the American Academy of Family Physicians, offered these thoughts: "Retail clinics are a manifestation of an entrepreneurial society taking advantage of a dysfunctional health care system. If we had a strong primary health care foundation in this country, you would not need retail clinics. With that said, retail clinics could be an important adjunct to primary care. They could help primary care extend their capacity and accessibility through extended hours."[65]

So, when considering primary care options, you may wish to look beyond the doctor's office. When the needs are simple and straightforward, your destination may be as close as the nearest Wal-Mart.

WHAT CAN YOU DO TO PROTECT YOUR HEALTH? STEP-BY-STEP ADVICE ON HOW TO FIND THE GOOD APPLES

We've broadly defined a set of criteria for helping evaluate physicians, beginning with your primary care doctor. Now let's get even more granular—down to the very questions you may wish to ask when seeking to discern which doctor is right for you.

Step 1: Finding the Right Primary Care Physician to Orchestrate Your Care and Understanding Why This Decision Is Critically Important

Imagine navigating the Amazon without a guide. Though the health care system isn't rife with venomous snakes and flesh-eating fish, there are a great many hazards that can make the experience torturous, expensive, and even deadly. Your tour guide, the one who keeps you out of harm's way, is your PCP. He or she has drawn the map for your journey, enlisted others to help you surmount obstacles, and carefully tracked your progress. When you need someone with specialized knowledge, your PCP should know the best resources to call on for help. When an unexpected complication arises, he or she knows how to course correct.

It's doubtful that you will find the Indiana Jones of primary care. What you will find, with a dedicated search, is a highly competent and compassionate physician who is dedicated to your family's health. You can improve your odds of finding the right PCP through a well-organized search process that includes some or all of the following elements.

Your search starts here:

- Decide whether it is important for your physician to adhere to a certain demographic profile:

  - Does it matter whether your physician is male or female?
  - Do you want your physician to fall within a certain age range?
  - Do you have any feelings relative to the ethnicity of your physician?

- As we've discussed, physicians undergo varying levels and types of education and training. It is important to identify what level of training and credentials are important to you:

  - Are you seeking a physician who has trained at a traditional medical school, or are you equally comfortable with someone who has undergone osteopathic training? There are subtle philosophical differences between the traditions that still exist today. You may find one more appealing than the other.

- How important is it that your physician be American trained? An increasing number of PCPs are foreign medical graduates. Their training may be impeccable, but it is a factor worthy of your consideration.
- Will you be more comfortable with a family-practice physician (who integrates care for patients of both genders and every age and who advocates for the patient in a complex health care system[66]) or with an internal-medicine physician (who provides long-term, comprehensive care, managing both common and complex illness of adolescents, adults, and the elderly[67])? If you select a family practice physician, what range of services are you comfortable receiving from this physician before being referred to a specialist (e.g., would you allow your FP to perform a colonoscopy, or would you expect to be referred to a gastroenterologist? What about delivering your baby?)?
- Do you value certain training institutions more than others, be it for medical school, osteopathic school, or residency? Would you, for instance, have higher confidence in an internist who trained at the Mayo Clinic?
- Is your physician board certified or board eligible by either the American Academy of Family Practice or the American Board of Internal Medicine?

- How will you determine whether your physician possesses the requisite experience, knowledge, and wisdom to manage your care optimally?

  - How many years has your physician been in practice?
  - How long has he or she been in their current practice?
  - What does your physician do to stay current on medical advancements? Can you discern whether they are a "lifelong learner?"
  - Can you obtain informed opinions from other physicians about your PCP?

- Have you been introduced to any of your PCP's partners—particularly the primary physician providing coverage when your physician is off or unavailable?
- What have you heard from friends and family about this physician? They may have limited ability to discern his or her clinical skills, but they may provide wonderful insight into the physician's bedside manner.

- Consider your physician's sphere of influence:

  - Are you comfortable with the hospital(s) with which your PCP is aligned? Since chances are you won't see him or her if hospitalized (hospitalists increasingly act as the primary care providers within the confines of the hospital), you should give this issue serious consideration.
  - Is your physician independent or employed by the hospital? If they are employed, all the more reason to be comfortable with that facility or system, since it may pressure your physician to use the resources of that system.
  - Your PCP may have a relatively tight-knit group of referral sources who are also tied to one or more hospitals. Are you familiar with some of the key specialists on whom your PCP relies, and are you comfortable with these groups based on your limited knowledge about them?

- Is the physician's philosophy of care congruent with your beliefs and values?

  - Under what circumstances would your physician consider it essential to see you the same day?
  - Does the physician welcome you as a collaborator in your care, or does he or she prefer that you defer to their judgment?
  - Is the physician relaxed and thorough when addressing your questions or concerns?
  - How does the physician manage your fear or anxiety? Is it with compassion, or is he or she dismissive?
  - How will your physician actively coordinate your care when multiple specialists may be involved?

- Does your physician have a particular bias toward medications in general or specific categories of drugs?
- How much importance does your physician place on wellness and prevention versus intervention? How do they demonstrate their commitment to wellness?
- How much importance does your physician place on well-being or emotional health? How do they demonstrate their commitment to this element of our lives?
- Does your physician practice within a medical home?
- Does your physician's staff include advance-practice nurses and nurse educators who can play an important role in your health?
- What is your physician's perspective on end-of-life care?

- How confident are you that your physician will recommend treatment regimens based on the latest medical science?

  - Does he or she practice evidence-based medicine?
  - Does he or she utilize an electronic medical record?
  - Are there standard protocols of care integrated into the record that your doctor relies on?

- Can you discern any other important information about your physician from trustworthy third-party data sources?

You can glean some of this information by scheduling an appointment to meet your potential new PCP and conduct an interview.

With perseverance complemented with a little luck, you will end up with the guide you need. Remember, though, even the best of guides are human. Your job is not to place blind trust in any single individual within the health care system but to use your discernment to know when to be deferential and when to seek more information. A good PCP will not be offended or threatened by your questions but, rather, respect your stewardship of your own health.

If you are worried about asking your doctors tough questions, get over it. As Charles Inlander advises, "the bottom line is that you have to walk in with an arsenal of questions to be able to pick a primary care doctor or specialist."[68] When we began, I indicated that selecting the right PCP is a formidable task. If you've done the homework, you are in agreement that the effort is well worth the time.

Otis Brawley, MD, offered similar advice when I asked him how a consumer could find the right physician, be it a PCP or specialist. "I think that people should interview doctors," he advises. "If someone has a chronic disease, this may be the most important interview of their life. Think of it as a hiring decision."[69]

Step 2: Selecting a Specialist When Needed

All patients, at some point, will need to see a specialist. When you do, your quest for information begins again in earnest. Start, of course, with your PCP—seek to ascertain why they are recommending a particular individual. Many of the questions that you asked of your PCP are relevant here. You should certainly understand the training, certification, and experience of the referred physician. If the referred specialist practices at the same health system as your PCP, additional due diligence may be required.

Though you would like to believe that he or she is godlike, in truth your PCP is exquisitely human. His or her recommendations for a specialist could be predicated on a host of reasons, including the following:

- Based on their experience with the specialist, your PCP is confident that you will get exemplary care from the recommended specialist. The PCP has your best interests in mind, though there may be blind spots in their assessment of the specialist's capabilities.
- Your PCP's sphere of influence is limited to the cadre of physicians aligned with his or her primary hospital, and thus he or she is not confident making a referral to someone outside the system.
- Your PCP is concerned about losing control of your care by referring you outside his or her sphere of influence. This is a common and realistic fear at times, particularly when community PCPs send their patients to specialists aligned with academic medical centers. Historically, these centers have been like black holes— attracting patients and then never allowing them to escape their gravitational force. Most academic centers are becoming more enlightened today—realizing that it is in everyone's best interest

to return the patient to the care of his or her community providers as soon as possible.
- The PCP is under significant pressure to keep referrals within the system. Health system management likely regards referrals to specialists outside the system as unnecessary losses in precious revenue it would otherwise capture.

Health systems want to capture all the specialty referrals possible from their PCPs (a large part of the reason why they employ PCPs). When PCPs aligned with a given system refer to specialists outside the system, it is referred to as *leakage*. Some health systems go to great lengths to stem such leakage. While hospitals or systems cannot mandate where a doctor sends his or her patients, they can make it uncomfortable to leak specialty referrals.

Some health systems, however, have a very different philosophy regarding leakage. Saint Luke's Health System, a Baldrige Award–winning health care system in Kansas City, employs hundreds of physicians, including a very large cadre of PCPs. Like other major health systems, there is often significant leakage out of the system (referrals going to nonaligned physicians), costing Saint Luke's millions of dollars each year.

Rather than exert influence or pressure on the employed PCPs in an effort to stem this leakage, former CEO Rich Hastings maintained a policy that specialists should win referrals. Hastings believed that PCPs should send their patients to whomever they perceived to offer the very best care. He hoped that it would be to doctors within his system, but he consistently put the patients' interest ahead of the bottom line of his health system. That's exactly what you should expect of your hospital and your PCP.

Though your selection of a specialist may begin with your PCP, it does not need to end there. Consider conducting your own investigation to ferret out the very best physician for your particular condition. Though much of the information you will unearth may be anecdotal, it is nonetheless grist for the mill of your decision-making process. When the same name comes up time and again in your search for the holy grail of specialty medicine, perhaps there's a reason for it.

Don't be overly impressed with titles, advises Otis Brawley, MD, indicating that people are often drawn to a specialist because he or she is the director or chief of a given service: "Quite honestly, these are frequently the doctors you want to avoid because their administrative responsibilities may mean they have little time for you." He then humbly added, "I've been a chief of service; I generally try to avoid them in my health care."[70]

Your first appointment with the specialist should provide a wealth of additional information. Many of the same screens you used with your PCP apply equally well with specialists, beginning with their education and certifications. Just as you assessed the fit with your PCP, you must be comfortable with this physician and his or her diagnosis and treatment plan. *If you have any doubts, even if based purely on intuition, it's time to get a second opinion.* Many experts would argue that there is always a benefit to getting additional opinions before proceeding with any significant intervention.

If you have any concerns about licensing or disciplinary actions taken against your physician, you may want to check out DocFinder, a website providing rapid access to most state boards, which allows you to view past disciplinary action by provider.[71]

Once you arrive at a decision regarding a specialist, be certain that your PCP is in the loop and supports your decision.

If your specialist recommends a procedure, get ready to roll up your sleeves; there's more information to dig out:

- Begin with a thorough understanding of the benefits and risks associated with the procedure.
- If undergoing surgery, determine the frequency with which your specialist performs the given procedure, as well as the experience the hospital staff has in managing patients with your diagnosis.
- Do not hesitate to ask about outcomes—both the specialist's and the hospital's.
- If the procedure involves anesthesia, you should have a clear understanding of (1) who will be administering the anesthesia, (2) what type of anesthesia will be used, and (3) what the risks are.
- What precautions will the facility take in the unlikely event a problem arises? Are there other options with lower risks and comparable benefits?
- Demand to know the complete costs of the planned procedure, as well as your personal obligation for the portion of the payment not

covered by insurance. You may wish to seek comparative-cost information if you believe that there are multiple providers of comparable quality in your market, particularly for lower-intensity interventions.

Heed Dr. Otis Brawley's sage advice: "As one of my favorite surgeons, Charlie Staley of Emory, likes to say, 'You only get one chance to do the surgery right, so choose your surgeon well, and pray you have an exceptional surgeon having an exceptionally good day.'"[72]

MYTH 6
"THERE'S NO BETTER PLACE TO BE WHEN YOU ARE ILL THAN THE HOSPITAL"

Try telling that to Willy King, a diabetic patient who had the wrong leg amputated during surgery. Was he the victim of an incompetent physician or a systemic failure of the system?

According to an article in the New York Times, "The blackboard to which surgeons refer in the operating room at University Community Hospital in Tampa listed the wrong leg for amputation, as did the operating room schedule and the hospital computer system, testimony revealed. By the time, Dr. Sanchez entered the operating room, the wrong leg had been sterilized and draped for surgery."[1] Mr. King's fate may well have been sealed with even the finest surgeon.

If you are thinking that King was the unfortunate one in a million, think again. The Joint Commission on Accreditation of Hospitals reported that cases of "wrong-site surgery" are frequent occurrences, happening as often as forty times per week.[2] If you are surprised by this alarming statistic, there's a great deal more you need to know about hospitals before ever setting foot in one. Before we embark on that journey, however, let me share a bit about my journey of discovery with hospitals.

MY EARLY INFATUATION WITH HOSPITALS

I started working in hospitals when I was sixteen, serving as an apprentice to the medical photographer at a major urban medical center. Our days were incredibly varied—shooting photomicroscopy slides in pathology one day, then scrubbing in to surgery to film a complex operation the next. As we crisscrossed many departments, I found myself in awe of the size and complexity of the organization. My mentor was not only incredibly talented at his job but also a wonderful tour guide who helped kindle my life-long interest in our health care delivery system.

One major element was lacking, however, from my many months spent in medical photography: there was very little exposure to patient care. So I volunteered to do a tour of duty as an orderly in the ER. It was one continuous adrenaline rush as nurses, physicians, and orderlies scurried like startled ants to address the emergent needs of our patients.

These experiences left me eager to learn more about these powerful institutions. But before that could happen, I needed to go to college, spread my wings, and determine the future course of my life. It would be nearly a decade, and by a very circuitous path, before I returned to work with hospitals.

PIERCING THE VEIL

In 1982, I was growing increasingly restless working for my family's retail firm. Though it was a highly successful, third-generation business, it held little interest for me. Against my father's strong advice, I decided to leave the firm and set out on my own to establish a strategic-marketing organization. My father's parting words of encouragement were "You'll starve."

Fortunately, time proved him wrong. However, I quickly realized that, as a twenty-five-year-old with no demonstrable experience outside my family's business, I had a tough road ahead. I had to find an emerging niche where no firm could claim a wealth of experience, or I might well starve! Fortuitously, hospital marketing was just coming into vogue, and I went after it with a vengeance.

With perseverance fueled by the angst of looming potential failure, I knocked and knocked and knocked on the doors of local hospitals until one finally gave me a chance to work my magic. That hospital happened to be the most highly regarded facility in our market, and one where I had no familial or other ties. Six months later, the hospital engaged my fledgling firm to manage all its health care marketing needs—a relationship that flourished for many years.

Over the next decade, my firm grew dramatically. As a result, I would have the privilege of working with hospital executives, physicians, and other health care providers across the nation. In the early years, my view of hospitals remained untarnished. These were hallowed institutions where the expertise of physicians combined with the latest medical technologies to rescue patients from the abyss—or so I thought.

As I developed closer relationships with hospital executives, I became privy to the challenges that kept them awake at night, which generally had little to do with marketing. Rather, they would be bedeviled by such things as inexplicably high rates of postoperative infections or the financial performance of failing departments. It did not take long for my naïveté to give way to an increasingly realistic assessment of the trials and tribulations of hospital executives.

As my awareness grew, my interests began to shift from addressing the marketing challenges of these organizations to the far greater challenge of identifying and addressing their core strategic issues. John Leifer, Ltd., a pioneering health care marketing firm, morphed into the Leifer Group, a strategic-planning organization. This transformation—or, in marketing speak, brand repositioning—began with the launch of a provocative publication known as *The Leifer Report*.

During its publication, *The Leifer Report* was regarded as a venue for thought-provoking dialogue regarding critical issues within the health care industry. It brought together highly divergent views on cutting-edge topics. Among the many contributors to *The Leifer Report* were President Bill Clinton; Speaker Newt Gingrich; Senators John Kerry and Paul Tsongas; Humana cofounder David Jones; integrative-medicine gurus Deepak Chopra, Andrew Weil, and Herbert Benson; and Pulitzer Prize–winning author Walt Bogdanich.

WALT BOGDANICH STRIPPED ME OF MY INNOCENCE

Walt Bogdanich is a tough, talented investigative journalist. In 1991 he published *The Great White Lie: How America's Hospitals Betray Our Trust and Endanger Our Lives* and in the span of three hundred–plus pages meticulously documented the spectacular failures of our modern hospitals—including one not far from my home.

Bogdanich's book eviscerated any remaining shreds of naïveté that I clung to regarding the impeccability of American hospitals. I was so taken with the power of his investigative reporting that I asked Bogdanich to write an article for *The Leifer Report*. Knowing that I was a consultant to the hospital industry, Bogdanich asked me if I was crazy—suggesting that promoting his ideas could be deleterious to my consulting career. I told him that I was happy to run that risk.

Here's a short quote from the article he wrote at my request:

> For fifteen years, I've been reporting on substandard hospitals and doctors. Their responses to my stories haven't changed a bit over time. "Anecdotes," they say, as if that somehow excuses the tragic, unnecessary loss of human life. To some degree, I expect this defensiveness—what professions, after all, are willing to readily admit their failings? I am more troubled by the widespread belief among politicians and patient consumers that bad medical care isn't a major problem.
>
> The phrase "Americans have the best medical care in the world" has been repeated so often by so many people that it has kept us from aggressively pursuing the question "How can we make it better?"[3]

A TIME-TESTED PERSPECTIVE

After thirty years of working within the health care industry, I can assure you that Bogdanich's observations were fair. The hospital industry is littered with case studies illustrating its dysfunction—from egregious errors to benign neglect. These are not rare events but daily occurrences in the life of American hospitals. As we shall see, these problems are not so much an issue of "bad" doctors or nurses but, rather, terribly flawed processes.

I would be remiss not to thank Bogdanich for planting a seed in me decades ago that is finally germinating in the form of this book. Like Bogdanich, my intent is not to cast aspersions on the industry but to lift the veil so that a resonant cry for change can ring as never before.

BACK TO BASICS: THE EVOLUTION OF THE AMERICAN HOSPITAL

Just as modern physicians have evolved from barber "surgeons," American hospitals have evolved from their earliest days as almshouses for the poor into highly complex organizations employing an armamentarium of advanced medical technology. This evolution can be seen in Bellevue Hospital Center, which began in 1736 as a mere six-bed ward within the New York City Almshouse and today treats approximately thirty thousand inpatients annually.[4]

As medical knowledge and technology advanced, so too did the American hospital. Today hospitals take on many forms as they strive to meet the diverse needs of patients across the nation.

THIRTY-ONE FLAVORS OF HOSPITALS

The evolution of our hospitals resulted in facilities of many "flavors." Since one of our goals is to ultimately discern which health care resources best fit our needs, it is important to understand the defining characteristics that differentiate these facilities—beginning with their areas of clinical focus or expertise.

The majority of hospitals are *general, acute-care* facilities. Translated, that means that they offer a broad array of services designed to meet most urgent or emergent care needs of the population they serve. At the other end of the spectrum are *specialty* hospitals, which provide a very narrow and focused range of services designed to serve a specific patient population. Examples of specialty hospitals include children's hospitals, mental health facilities, and dedicated heart or orthopedic hospitals.

Both general and specialty care hospitals vary dramatically by *size*— with a common unit of measure being the number of staffed beds (a measure of inpatient capacity). Small rural hospitals may have as few as ten beds, whereas major urban centers can exceed a thousand. As one would naturally assume, the breadth and depth of services generally correlates with size.

Within the industry, the relative *sophistication* of hospitals is delineated by ascribing one of four levels of care: primary, secondary, tertiary, and quaternary. A primary care facility is extremely limited in services, whereas a quaternary facility offers cutting-edge treatment modalities that may include transplant services, burn centers, neonatal intensive care units, and other "high-acuity" services. Complexity, however, should not be regarded as any guarantee of quality, safety, or value of the care delivered by these institutions.

Most quaternary hospitals are *academic* facilities, which differ in important ways from *community* hospitals. As academic facilities, they have a tripartite mission, which includes the provision of care, the teaching of physicians, and the deepening of knowledge through medical research. Their physicians are generally on staff and salaried, whereas community physicians historically have been independent entrepreneurs, often practicing at multiple hospitals. In academic settings, patients are often cared for by a combined team of physicians, including an attending (a supervising physician) and a resident (a physician in training).

Hospitals also vary based on their sponsorship, with the simplest division being between *faith-based* and *secular* facilities. Though faith-based hospitals dominated America for centuries, there has been an increasing trend toward secularization in recent years.

A sharper contrast may be seen between *for-profit* and *not-for-profit* hospitals. The majority of hospitals in America are not-for-profit facilities. The term *not-for-profit* is a reference to the entity's tax designation. It has little bearing on the hospital's actual financial performance. Up until recently, "margins" of 5 to 10 percent were not uncommon among not-for-profits in the industry, despite efforts by payers to ratchet down hospital reimbursement.

What do hospitals do with this money? Their not-for-profit status obligates the hospital to use any financial benefit accrued in a way that furthers it mission and benefits the patients served.

For-profit hospitals, which prefer the term *tax-paying*, are in the business of generating a return on investment to their shareholders. In his book *A Second Opinion* Arnold Relman, MD, professor emeritus at Harvard Medical School and editor emeritus of the *New England Journal of Medicine*, shared these findings about for-profit hospitals:

- One careful study in 2002 reviewed all the available published data for U.S. private for-profit and not-for-profit hospitals, pooled the results, and found that the risk of patient death was 2 percent higher in the for-profit hospitals.[5]
- An interesting report in 1999 compared Medicare spending in geographic areas in which all acute-care hospitals were for-profit with spending in areas in which all the hospitals were not-for-profit. Adjusted mean per capita Medicare spending on inpatient care, as well as total spending, was much higher in the for-profit area, and spending rose when all not-for-profit hospitals in an area were converted to for-profit ownership.[6]

In fairness to for-profit hospitals, it should be noted that many industry observers see little difference, beyond an IRS designation, between the behavior of for-profit hospitals and not-for-profit facilities. Even so, I adhere to the adage, *What is good for Wall Street is not necessarily good for Main Street.*

Finally, hospitals may either be *stand-alone* facilities or members of a *health care system.* The largest for-profit health care system is HCA—Hospital Corporation of America—with more than 160 hospitals in twenty states. The largest not-for-profit system is Ascension Health, a Catholic system serving more than fifteen hundred locations.

THREE POINTS OF COMMONALITY

Regardless of their important points of differentiation, I would argue that there are three defining characteristics shared by the majority of American hospitals:

- they are dangerous,
- they are horrifically expensive, and
- they are not customer-focused.

What underlies such dysfunction? In a word, *variation.*

VARIATION: THE ROOT OF MOST DYSFUNCTION

In any industry, there is universal agreement that variation destroys the efficiency of a smoothly operating factory while simultaneously raising the costs of production—whether it is an auto-assembly line or a hospital, which should function like a smoothly operating factory of care.

Much of what we know about the impact of variation comes from the pioneering work of W. Edwards Deming. Deming was a statistician who spent the early years of his career working in post–World War II Japan. At the time, any product bearing the sticker "Made in Japan" was perceived to be of inferior quality. This attitude was not merely residual resentment from the war but testimony to the level of variation in many of Japan's manufacturing plants.

Deming realized that, if Japan were to transform its war-ravaged economy into a modern industrial nation, it would have to address this problem and eliminate the associated stigma. So he began teaching Japanese engineers the principles of statistical process control, which would allow them to significantly bolster the quality of manufactured goods.[7]

Nowhere was the impact of Deming's transformative approach more apparent than in the Japanese automotive industry. Over several decades, it went from producing cars with highly variable and questionable quality to being the worldwide leader in quality and dependability. Deming demonstrated that controlling variation is essential to achieving efficiency and quality. It was the difference between a cottage industry producing one-off products and a smoothly operating factory producing a remarkably consistent product.

Deming had such a profound impact on the Japanese economy that he came to be viewed as a national treasure. In 1960 "he was awarded the Order of the Sacred Treasure, second class, the highest Japanese award ever given to foreigners."[8] The award was bestowed on him by the emperor.

Deming was frequently quoted as saying, "If I had to reduce my message for management to just a few words, I'd say it all had to do with reducing variation." The world's greatest authority on process standardization taught us that this universal principle applies equally to hospitals and to the auto industry.

Thus, in a perfect world, hospitals would be capable of producing standardized outcomes with tremendous efficiency. Though hospitals are taking steps toward the minimization of variation in their processes, the pace of change is glacial at a time when it needs to be explosively transformational.

The variation that occurs within and across hospitals manifests in many ways. Its symptoms include everything from dramatic differences in postsurgical mortality rates to widely disparate costs. Why is there so much variation in health care? One reason is the complexity of medicine. There are virtually infinite variations in patient presentation, making it difficult to engineer standardized care protocols for all conditions

WHAT HOSPITALS COULD LEARN FROM McDONALD'S

Before delving deeper, let's take a short side trip to a non-health care company that understands the extraordinary importance of minimizing variation in processes.

No one understands this lesson better than the executives at McDonald's. There is much that they could teach the health care industry! Don't worry; the lessons we are going to glean from McDonald's are not about nutrition. Rather, they are about maintaining consistency in quality while maximizing efficiency.

McDonald's serves well over fifty million people daily in 120 countries worldwide. It generates more than $20 billion in revenue and enjoys a strong profit margin. It maintains its global success based on consistency, which translates into predictability for consumers. A quarter pounder in Washington, D.C., tastes the same as one in Wellington, New Zealand.

McDonald's has achieved this consistency by creating the smoothly operating factory of food. Extremely tight process engineering ensures not only uniformity in the product but also extraordinary efficiency—which translates into value for its customers and shareholders. It maintains these standards through training, with nearly three hundred thousand people having graduated from McDonald's Hamburger University.

Whereas safety issues are endemic in health care, such problems are a rarity in McDonald's. The company, which could easily fall prey to the safety issues associated with contaminated food, avoids such problems by infusing its restaurants and suppliers with a culture of safety. Each restaurant must conduct seventy-two daily safety-protocol checks. All beef suppliers must comply with quality and safety testing every two hours. Even potato providers go through ninety-five daily safety/quality checks.

Now imagine for a moment what McDonald's would be like if the food quality varied dramatically between restaurants. What if there were no prices posted on its menus? What if the prices varied tremendously from location to location? How would you feel waiting for hours to receive your order? And, finally, what if you had to worry about the safety of your food each time you visited McDonald's?

It's hard to imagine McDonald's flourishing under such conditions. Yet that's exactly the type of variation we find within health care. Health care is the antithesis of the smoothly operating factory. It is far more like a cottage industry with little standardization. As we have now seen, there is variability in the frequency with which various procedures are used, the quality of those procedures, and their associated costs, all topics we will continue to explore in greater detail.

TREATING PATIENTS IS NOT AS EASY AS FLIPPING BURGERS

Imagine for a moment that two patients simultaneously arrive in the ER of a busy hospital, complaining of unremitting chest pain. A quick, standardized diagnostic workup indicates that both patients are in the throes of a heart attack. The first patient is otherwise quite healthy and had been out for a run shortly before being stricken with painful symptoms. He may be treated using a standardized protocol involving the administration of a clot-busting drug known as TPA. Once the acute episode is under control and he is out of danger, other interventions, including angioplasty, will be considered.

The second patient is far more complex. He has four major underlying conditions (referred to in the industry as comorbidities), including diabetes, high blood pressure, chronic obstructive pulmonary disease, and coronary-artery disease. He is the proverbial train wreck, and, adding insult to injury, the ER doctors learn that the patient has undergone multiple angioplasties in the past in attempts to prevent the very heart attack that is happening at that moment. These factors make this patient's course of treatment far more complex and thus less amenable to standardization.

Soon a host of specialists is assembled to consult on the patient's condition. Each doctor has a slightly different view as to the most appropriate next steps in treating the patient. None of the doctors is "wrong," because the evidence supporting specific interventions in such cases is either lacking or equivocal. As the complexity of the patient's condition increases, so too do the number of consulting physicians, and the level of potential variation in care grows astronomically

ADDITIONAL FACTORS DRIVING VARIATION

The second major factor complicating efforts at standardization of care is the stunning lack of comparative evidence regarding the most efficient and effective methods of treating many conditions, as described in chapter 3. Hospitals do have pathways designed to minimize care variation for a variety of conditions. But there are countless conditions for which such clinical templates do not exist. Furthermore, the existence of such pathways is no guarantee of their usage by the medical staff.

A third major factor driving variation can be seen in the manner in which hospitals manage their finances. The incomprehensible variation seen in hospital charges is a symptom of broad variation in the levels of discounts contractually provided to insurers, the manner in which fixed costs are assigned, and other factors that we will examine shortly. Thus prices fluctuate widely.

A fourth factor driving variation is greed. Some physicians may deliver interventions that do not conform to standards of care but do serve to line their pockets. Hospital administrators can easily turn a blind eye because it is not within their domain to question the clinical judgment of the medical staff unless they happen to be a peer.

Perhaps the most important factor driving variation in hospitals is "culture." For a large number of American hospitals, gross variation in processes seems to be accepted as an unavoidable aspect of care. These organizations are more focused on economics than on finding transformational solutions that help render far more efficient and effective outcomes.

THE 5 PERCENT SOLUTION

Five percent of hospitals are outliers in a positive sense. They do things very differently from the norm.

The 5 percent minority may have much to teach us about care. Organizations like the Mayo Clinic demonstrate that high levels of process standardization are achievable and that superlative affordable care is often the result. What drives Mayo? A culture in which minimization of variation in process, coupled with clinical and service excellence as measured by outcomes and efficiency, are the organization's raison d'être. It's also an institution that has strictly controlled physicians' salaries. Doctors practice there because they are motivated by far more than "mere" money.

THE COMPLEXITY OF CARE COORDINATION ACROSS PROVIDERS

It is essential to remember that most care is delivered outside the hospital. In fact, the majority of it is delivered in physicians' offices, where such pathways may be nonexistent. Even in the presence of clinical guidelines, many physicians continue to practice largely as they were taught. We know that there is significant variation in teaching programs and that medical knowledge becomes outdated very quickly.

Health care services are also delivered in ambulatory-delivery sites, remote imaging centers, outpatient-surgery facilities, radiation centers, nursing homes, and so forth. If we are to standardize care processes, we must achieve phenomenal coordination across this broad, disconnected care enterprise.

That may sound easy, but it is a Herculean task. Think for a moment about what that would require:

- One physician, presumably the primary care physician, would need to be the quarterback—calling the plays that allow the patient to utilize all these disparate services in an appropriate and timely fashion. The doctor's actions would be based on scientifically reliable data supporting every test or intervention, not intuition, nor influence by clinical "noise."

- As specialists are brought into the case, these physicians, who are likely to be at separate delivery sites, would need to understand the nuances of the patient's condition in order to render the optimal result. Hence, they would need easy access to a comprehensive patient record, which they would then update upon concluding their work. Their interventions, whether diagnostic or treatment, would also be predicated on the latest scientific data.

- With each new physician encounter, the patient's condition, prognosis, and need for potential modifications to the treatment plan may become evident, requiring the primary physician (quarterback) to stay in the game and adjust the care plan on the fly.

- Since some of the recommended tests or treatments may be questioned by insurance companies wanting to avoid unnecessary costs, the physicians must run interference with case managers and be prepared to provide a strong rationale for their recommended care.

- Each new drug given to the patient would need to be screened for possible synergistic effects with drugs prescribed by other doctors. If the patient is to undergo certain procedures, the taking of some drugs, such as blood-thinning agents, would need to be suspended.

- Since patients' records are currently a hodgepodge of paper and electronic files, there would need to be a single, electronic repository for this information that would facilitate real-time access by all the caregivers.

- If the patient's condition deteriorates to the point where they have to be hospitalized, a new cadre of caregivers would need to be integrated—including hospitalists and nurses.

- Throughout this process, the patient and his or her family would need to be kept informed in order to participate in shared decision making with their providers.

An entire army of Six Sigma Black Belts could not engineer their way out of this dilemma. Minimization of variation across these disparate providers would require a very different care model than exists in the market today.

Don Berwick, former secretary of Health and Human Services, summed it up nicely when he said that "such undesirable variation derives, for example, from misinterpretation of random noise in clinical data, from unreliability in the performance of clinical and support systems intended to support care, from habitual differences in practice style that are not grounded in knowledge or reason, and from the failure to integrate care across the boundaries or components of the health care system."[9]

Now that we know a bit about why variation occurs, let's take a look at its impact in greater detail.

VARIATION IN QUALITY OF CARE

It doesn't take a rocket scientist to discern that the variance in quality between hospitals is striking—even across disciplines within a given hospital. There are reams of data supporting this assertion—enough to fill books, if not libraries. This data comes in the form of peer-reviewed studies, such as one that appeared in the October 2009 edition of the *New England Journal of Medicine*. Its authors, Ghaferi et al., examined the level of "Variation in Hospital Mortality Associated with Inpatient Surgery."[10]

Their study was extensive. The authors examined, in detail, nearly eighty-five thousand surgical patients over a two-year period—as well as the events after surgery. They determined that, though the rates for postsurgical complications were statistically comparable across hospitals in the study, the mortality associated with these complications varied dramatically. "Patients who were treated at very-high-mortality hospitals had nearly two times the likelihood of dying after the development of a major complication as did their counterparts in very-low-mortality hospitals (21.4 percent vs. 12 percent, $p < 0.001$)."[11]

The Dartmouth Atlas provides another source of data examining variations in quality across hospitals. The website began publishing a new report in 2012 that examines quality-related metrics at twenty-three teaching hospitals. "The list demonstrates that even hospitals with excellent reputations may fall short in certain quality measures, said Dr. David Goodman, a principal investigator on the Atlas project."[12]

A hospital may boast an excellent heart program and have the data to prove it. Excellence in one area is no guarantee of quality in another. Through astute marketing, hospital executives leverage a point of differentiation, successfully convincing consumers that the halo of excellence associated with the heart program extends across all their services, despite being clinically deficient in many areas.

THE DANGER LURKING IN AMERICA'S HOSPITALS

Perhaps the most startling revelation about hospitals is the degree to which they imperil patient safety. We began this segment by looking at one example of a hospital-induced injury. Allow me to share a few more tales—including one that I personally witnessed.

Tragedy Strikes at One of America's Finest Hospitals: Downing a Rising Star

Harvard-affiliated teaching hospitals symbolize the strength of American medicine.[13] Among these giants, one in particular stands out—Massachusetts General Hospital. It was here, in 1846, that the public witnessed the miracle of the first painless surgery performed under anesthesia.

There have been many firsts at Mass General—often bringing renewed promises of life where before there had been little hope for desperately ill patients. But like all hospitals, Mass General has witnessed its share of tragedies, including ones that were avoidable.

In the tough world of television production, there are also giants, and Trevor Nelson was well on his way to becoming one. Though only thirty-four years old, he had already made his mark in the industry as a producer of the award-winning program 60 Minutes. Though his job was demanding, he always found time for what was most precious—his family.

While on vacation with his wife, Maggie, and sons, George and Conrad, Nelson became ill. Though he tried to ignore it, he couldn't shake the headache that accompanied his general sense of malaise, driving him to seek treatment at a local hospital. A short battery of test revealed little about Nelson's condition, and he was discharged with medication. The medicine, however, proved to be of little help in ameliorating Nelson's wracking headache. So, three days later, Trevor and Maggie drove to the Mass General's ER. [14]

With more than eighty-five thousand visits per year, Mass General's ER bustles like a small city. The seasoned staff, who are accustomed to treating major trauma, not "mere" headaches, saw no reason for undue alarm. In fact, after a number of hours had passed, they suggested that Maggie return home to care for the boys. Reluctant to leave, Maggie finally acquiesced, accepting the staff's promises that her husband would be fine.

But Trevor was not fine. Diagnosed with non-life-threatening viral meningitis, Nelson was admitted to the hospital. During the course of his visit, he was given a plethora of powerful drugs to alleviate his intractable headache—purportedly including more than twelve doses of narcotics in fifteen hours. [15] *Early the next morning, when nurses came to check on him, they discovered he had no vital signs. Though placed on life support, Trevor Nelson would never recover . . . and nor would his family from their epic loss. Was his death attributable to a fatal combination of drugs that suppressed the central nervous system, as the family alleges . . . and was thus avoidable? That question would be determined by a jury.*

The Case of the Blazing Patient

There's nothing esoteric about an electrocautery. The device has been a fixture of virtually all operating rooms for nearly a century. As its name implies, electrocautery can be used to stem the flow of blood during surgery through cauterization of tissues and blood vessels. It can also be used to make an incision. In most situations it is both safe and invaluable.

There are exceptions, however, as "Mary," an eighteen-year-old patient undergoing emergency surgery for a ruptured appendix, was about to find out. As Mary was being prepared for surgery, her skin was treated first with iodine and then with an alcohol compound known as spirit. The initial incisions were made, and as the operation progressed, the surgeon began to cauterize the surgical site. Following is an account of what happened next.

> As soon as the cautery was used, the cotton wound towels applied on the two sides of the incision caught fire due to a flame arising from the undersurface of the towel. It was extinguished using another sponge but not before producing deep dermal burns on two sides of the skin incision. The cautery was checked and found to be correctly installed. On careful examination, it was observed that the skin was still wet with the last coating of spirit, which was not dried up properly. The residual spirit film on the skin caught fire from the spark of the cautery leading to burns involving the lower part of the anterior abdominal wall. It took three weeks for the deep dermal burns to heal with residual scarring. [16]

A research study published in the May 2013 issue of *Anesthesiology* examined the cause of OR fires using insurance-claims data. The researchers determined that the electrocautery was the source of ignition 90 percent of the time. [17] The most frequent cause was the ignition of oxygen being administered to anesthetized patients, though "alcohol-containing prep solutions and volatile compounds were present in . . . 15 percent of OR fires during monitored anesthesia." [18]

The Tragedy of Multiple Deaths Due to a Single Avoidable Error

Heparin is an extremely potent drug used to thin a patient's blood as a preventative for strokes and other adverse events. It is commonly used in neonatal intensive care units (NICUs) to keep the IV lines open in premature babies. The drug can be lifesaving when properly administered and lethal when given in the wrong dose.

On September 16, 2006, tragedy struck the NICU at Indianapolis-based Methodist Hospital, part of the Clarian health system (now IU Health). It began with a silent but deadly error—when vials of heparin containing adult doses of the drug were delivered inadvertently to the NICU by an experienced pharmacy tech. [19] With tens of thousands of prescriptions being filled each day by Clarian pharmacists, it simply slipped through the cracks. Though there were numerous times when the error might have been identified, no one caught it before the drugs were administered.

As a result, six babies received a dose of heparin that was one thousand times more powerful than prescribed.[20] Three of the babies died. Three were injured. As a consultant to the organization, I witnessed this tragedy unfold, albeit at some distance. I saw the ensuing anguish that cascaded through the organization. Everyone was heartbroken, as, of course, were the families of those tiny children.

The children were gone, and there was nothing the team at Clarian could do to change that fact. But, much to the credit of Clarian's administrative and physician leadership, they immediately went public with the painful truth behind the tragedy, promising that these tiny lives would not be sacrificed in vain. The team then devoted themselves to identifying and fixing the systemic breakdowns within their hospitals so that such tragedies would not be repeated.

A Mother Loses Her Precious Daughter

Desiree Wade was full of life. As a four-year-old girl, she dreamed of being a ballerina—dreams that helped shield her from the difficult reality of life in Harlem and brought joy into her life. When doctors suggested to her mother, Beverly, that Desiree needed a tonsillectomy, she assumed it was a minor operation with few risks. And she was right, in terms of statistical averages, but not in terms of the one outcome that mattered most to her—her precious daughter's health.

Desiree began to show symptoms of a problem the day after what appeared to have been an unremarkable surgery. Seventy-two hours later, Desiree was hemorrhaging massive amounts of blood from her mouth, dying shortly thereafter in her mother's arms.[21] A beautiful life, a mother's hopes and dreams, cut tragically short by a surgical complication arguably due to a poorly trained provider.

A Kidney Goes Missing

In August 2013, CNN broke a story regarding the University of Toledo Medical Center.[22] According to reporter John Bonifield, patient Sarah Fudacz was hospitalized for a kidney transplant. Her brother, Paul, was a perfect match. So on August 10 of 2012, Paul underwent surgery to remove one of his kidneys so that it could be transplanted into his sister.

The surgery went swimmingly. Unfortunately, though, a nurse inadvertently threw the kidney away. Hard to believe? It really happened. Dr. Jeffrey Gold, chancellor and executive vice president for Health Affairs at the university, offered a profound apology. The matter is now in the courts.[23]

THESE CASES ARE NOT ISOLATED EXAMPLES

As outlined in chapter 1, hospital-induced injuries, illness, and death are a major problem in the United States. The extent of health care's dirty laundry was fully exposed in 2000, when the Institute of Medicine (IOM) published, *To Err Is Human: Building a Safer Health Care System*. Headlines across the nation proclaimed that medical errors were now one of the leading causes of death in our nation.

The report was groundbreaking. The fact that such sensational findings came out of a methodical study conducted by the IOM made it difficult to refute, though plenty of pundits tried. Most importantly, though, "the report called for a fundamental transformation in the delivery of health care, emphasizing the culpability of the entire medical system rather than individual physicians."[24]

This report was akin to Upton Sinclair's 1906 book, *The Jungle*, which exposed the ills of the meatpacking industry, resulting in dramatic industry changes over time. Sinclair was a muckraking journalist. The IOM is a distinguished scientific body. If Sinclair could catalyze wholesale change across an industry, could not the IOM?

Despite the concussive effects of its initial publication, the IOM report does not appear to be having a dramatic impact on the safety of American hospitals. High rates of errors continue to plague our hospitals, based on the current research.

Hospital-induced errors were the key focus of *To Err Is Human*, but such errors are pervasive throughout the delivery system—from the physician's office to the ambulatory surgery center. Just how pervasive are errors within our health care system? A 2002 study revealed that "35 percent of physicians and 42 percent of the public reported errors in their own or a family member's care."[25]

According to Walshe and Shortell, hospitals have a long history of sweeping problems under the rug, thus preventing improvement in processes across the system. "It is striking," they say, "that major failures are not usually brought to light by the systems for quality assurance or improvement that are now found in most health care organization in developed countries."[26]

Walshe and Shortell reinforce their point by citing a somewhat dated but glaring example of this issue. "At Vermillion County Hospital in Indiana, where Orville Lynn Majors worked in intensive care and murdered patients, there were twenty-four deaths in the intensive care unit (ICU) in 1991, twenty-five in 1992, thirty-one in 1993, and 101 in 1994, but the quality-management systems did not identify a problem."[27]

Despite incredible pressure on hospitals to clean up their act, mistakes are still happening at an alarming rate. The May 5, 2013, online edition of the *St. Louis Post-Dispatch* reported the case of a fifty-three-year-old paralegal named Regina Turner.

Apparently, a neurosurgeon operating at St. Clare Health Center in Fenton, Missouri, operated on the wrong side of Ms. Turner's brain. As a result, according to Ms. Turner's attorney, the patient "now requires around-the-clock care and cannot speak intelligibly."[28]

A less malignant but nonetheless damaging form of error is the system's failure to provide the requisite services for its patients. The IOM published a book on quality and error, *Crossing the Quality Chasm*. In it Sarah Bleich concludes that "the average patient receives only 55 percent of the services that would benefit that individual," according to an IOM Report in 2001.[29]

In the automotive industry, there are extensive warranties on the product you are purchasing in order to provide a safeguard. In health care, not only are there no warranties, but providers stand to profit from the very problems they create through poor quality delivery.

PROFITING FROM ERROR VERSUS PROFITING FROM IMPROVEMENT

Hospitals have long had a perverse disincentive to eliminate error: They make money from it. Though the rules for Medicare patients have changed, many private payers still cover the additional costs associated with hospital-induced infections and injuries—so-called *iatrogenic events*.

Consider the findings of a recent study published in the *Journal of the American Medical Association* that examined the records of more than thirty-four thousand surgical patients treated by a Texas health care system. Among these patients, 1,820 experienced complications. Researchers found that "the median length of stay for those patients quadrupled to fourteen days, and hospital revenue averaged $30,500 more for patients without complications ($49,400 versus $18,900)."[30]

Shortly after the publication of *To Err Is Human*, I sat in numerous meetings with hospital executive teams from across the country. The lion's share of these teams seemed absolutely committed to seeking solutions to the problem of medical errors. Even so, more than once I encountered hospital executives who explained that the errors that I wanted to help them eliminate contributed to their hospital's bottom line. I was at a loss for words. In speaking with other consultants, I realized that such discussions were happening quietly in executive conference rooms across America.

The federal government, primarily through Medicare, is taking a big step forward in reducing inappropriate reimbursement for hospital-induced conditions. State government and private payers are also experimenting with models for eliminating this perverse incentive. When the state of Maryland created incentives based on reductions in HAIs— hospital-acquired infections—the resulting changes to hospital complication rates and costs were startling: "During the first two years that Maryland's incentive program was in place, complication rates declined by 15.2 percent, resulting in $110.9 million savings in the system, which equals 0.6 percent of total inpatient costs."[31]

DISCLOSING ERROR RATES

Transparency is an essential component when addressing the issue of medical error. Patients have a right to know whether their chosen hospital is safe. The government took steps to improving safety transparency but then capitulated to complaints from the industry and announced that the information would be pulled: "Two years ago, over objections from the hospital industry, the federal government announced it would add data about 'potentially life-threatening' mistakes made in hospitals to a website people can search to check on safety performance. Now, the Centers for Medicare and Medicaid Services plan to remove the eight hospital-acquired conditions, which include infections and mismatched blood transfusions, while it comes up with a different set."[32]

CMS's decision enraged a number of consumer groups and business coalitions across the nation that saw the withdrawal of this information as a step backward in the push for transparency. Can you imagine an airline that was allowed to cover up all its accidents regardless of how many lives had been lost or passengers injured?

It should be crystal clear by now that the care delivered by hospitals across the nation is highly variable in quality and safety, but what about the cost of care? If you are staggered by the variation in quality and safety, you will be floored by the variation in charges among hospitals.

DECIPHERING THE COST OF COMPLEX AND HIGHLY VARIABLE CARE

Steven Brill, in a methodically constructed exposé on our health care system that appeared in *Time* magazine, posed an essential question that health care reform has seemed to sidestep: "When we debate health care policy, we seem to jump right to the issue of who should pay the bills, blowing past what should be the first question: Why exactly are the bills so high?"[33]

Those bills can be staggering—amounting to tens if not hundreds of thousands of dollars for patients blindsided by the cost of their illness or injury. What can we discern about the costs of such care?

Close to one-third of our nation's $2.8 trillion health care bill is attributable to hospital costs—costs that have escalated at a staggering pace over the past three decades. "Overall spending for hospital services reached $814 billion in 2010."[34] It was $100 billion in 1980, $250 billion in 1990, and $415 billion in 2000.[35] Though consumers may have been aware of the heavy toll charged by hospitals, very few, until recently, were aware of the level of variation in charges among facilities, let alone how these prices are derived.

We've all heard about the proverbial $10 aspirin, but what about the $546 bag of saline? According to *New York Times* reporter Nina Bernstein, patients receiving a standard saline IV are often charged hundreds of dollars for a product that costs between fifty cents and a dollar to manufacture.[36]

The last time I checked, saltwater was not in short supply. There were oceans full of it. So how can hospitals justify such outrageous markups? That's a question all of us should be asking.

Thanks to the federal government's release of data on hospital charges, coupled with the publication of several exposés on the health care industry, awareness is changing. In May 2013, the Department of Health and Human Services (HHS) released data on hospital charges, in which they "highlighted variations in the undiscounted prices hospitals charge for the same procedures. Specifically, joint-replacement charges ranged from $5,300 at a hospital in Ada, Okla., to $223,000 charged at a hospital in Monterey Park, Calif."[37]

Perhaps you noted the term *undiscounted prices* in the HHS release. Hospitals use many terms to obscure the true price of their services. It is a complex game of chess played out between the provider of services and the purchaser. So before we can attempt to understand the level of variation in hospital prices, we must first understand how prices are derived. Our starting point will be a quasi–price list known as the hospital *charge master*.

RETAIL PRICES IN A WHOLESALE-ONLY WORLD

In health care, *charges* are the fictionalized fees that a provider would obtain in a world devoid of insurance or governmental discounts. They represent so-called retail fees in a wholesale-only world. Hospitals maintain a master list of their charges, referred to as a charge master (also known as *chargemaster*). No consideration is given to quality, safety, or outcome of the hospital's care when constructing the charge master.

Virtually every payer receives a discount from charges. The rates of discounts vary profoundly across hospitals and health systems, geographic markets, and insurance carriers. In markets where little to no competition exists for a hospital's business, purchasers have only a weak leg to stand on when negotiating rates.

Research published in 2006 found that "the gap between charges and actual payments (net patient revenues) now averages about 255 percent and is growing rapidly."[38]

Discounts can range upward of 80 percent. Steven Brill finds that "according to its latest financial report, Seton [Medical Center in Daly, California] applies so many discounts and write-offs to its chargemaster bills that it ends up with only about 18 percent of the revenue it bills. That's an average 82 percent discount, compared with an average discount of about 65 percent that I saw at the other hospitals whose bills were examined."[39] Brill goes on to say that, "no matter how steep the discounts, the chargemaster prices are so high and so devoid of any calculation related to cost that the result is uniquely American: thousands of nonprofit institutions have morphed into high-profit, high-profile businesses that have the best of both worlds."[40]

Since the charge master is largely illusionary to begin with, it is difficult to make cogent observations regarding the impact of this variation on value delivery across hospitals or markets.

There are no other industrialized nations hampered by this lack of true price transparency. In fact, in countries such as Japan, a national fee schedule is published that "sets forth exactly what a doctor, therapist, or hospital will be paid for any treatment or medication."[41]

How do our prices compare to those in Japan? "In the United States, a standard MRI scan of the head costs about $1,000 to $1,400. In Japan, the health ministry thinks that price is far too high. The fixed price for an MRI of the head in Japan is Y11,400 or $105."[42]

Before you conclude that the Japanese must suffer from inferior health or health care, you should know a couple of facts. By many measures, including longevity, the Japanese are the healthiest people on the planet. Remember that, though they are among the most aggressive consumers of health care, their national health care bill, as measured in terms of percentage of GDP, is a fraction of the U.S. bill.[43]

The charge master is opaque to consumers. Only the state of California requires that hospitals publish their charge masters online. Even if more broadly disseminated, publication would be of little value to consumers. Much as physicians use arcane terms to cloak their profession, hospitals use similar verbal sleight of hand to render their "true" prices virtually impenetrable. How much variability is there among charge masters? According to Brill, "No hospital's chargemaster prices are consistent with those of any other hospital, nor do they seem to be based upon anything objective—like cost—that any hospital executive I spoke with was able to explain."[44]

Once upon a time, many years ago, the charge master actually correlated with what it cost a hospital to produce a service. Today the listed charges have virtually no bearing on what the actual, direct cost of the service or product is to the hospital or what the hospital is ultimately paid. As Steven Brill succinctly concluded in his article on hospital billing, "there seems to be no process, nor rationale, behind the core document that is the basis for hundreds of billions of dollars in health care bills."[45]

Unraveling the truth behind the charge master becomes more complicated due to the multiplicity of unique purchasing agreements that hospitals negotiate with payers. Because hospitals enter into one-off contracts with payers that may have highly variable rates of discount from charges, the same procedure using the same charge master may result in significant variance in actual billed charges.

The level of discount accorded a payer is generally a function of the clout of the payer relative to that of the provider in a given market. A powerful health system that is highly regarded by consumers, and therefore perceived as essential to a payer's network of hospitals, would therefore have far more sway at the bargaining table than a stand-alone hospital of questionable reputation.

Does anyone pay full freight for their hospital stay? Tragically, the group most likely to pay full charges has been the one least able to afford it—the medically indigent who lack health insurance. Due to a public outcry at the hospital practice of billing full charges to the impoverished, most hospitals now bill at the "average discount rate" from charges.

It is the charge master, a tool unknown to virtually all Americans, that is arguably at the very core of our health care system's dysfunction. Consider the follwoing:

- "The charge master sits at the vortex of government regulation, rapidly growing health care costs, growing segments of the population lacking sufficient or any insurance, and enduring philosophical legacy of "optimizing reimbursement." The charge master might be an accounting tool, but its role reflects and, in turn, affects some of the deepest controversies and stressors in the U.S. health care system."[46]

- "For patients, the charge master are both the real and the metaphoric essence of the broken market. They are anything but irrelevant. They're the source of the poison coursing through the health care ecosystem."[47]

The Affordable Care Act may make health care far more accessible to millions, but it does not say a word in its more than two thousand pages about the charge master.

In 2012, a series of eight consumer focus groups addressing the issue of "transparency in health care" was conducted by the American Institutes for Research at the behest of the Robert Wood Johnson Foundation. The authors concluded that "consumers find information on the cost of care difficult to obtain and understand. They attribute these feelings to (a) the fragmented way in which they receive bills for different elements of their service (versus a single bill for an episode of care); (b) the tremendous costs for mundane consumer items, e.g., aspirin, creates cognitive dissonance . . . they don't understand; (c) no one helps to translate their bill."[48] There has to be a more equitable and transparent way of pricing hospital services!

HOSPITALS ARE THE ANTITHESIS OF VALUE-DRIVEN

In the absence of standardized quality, safety, and cost data, how does one have an intelligent discussion about the comparative value delivered by hospitals? Even if such data existed, there would still be disagreements as to what constitutes value. Like beauty, value is in the eye of the beholder. It may mean one thing to a patient and something very different to a payer.

Despite these obstacles, I believe it is essential to move toward an agreed-upon definition of value—beginning with the patient's perspective. The patient, after all, is the consumer of the care. They are also bearing an increasing burden for the cost of that care. If patients are uniform and resolute in their demands for value, they will possess tremendous power—whether lobbying their employers to make value-based purchasing decisions, bringing pressure on providers, or challenging their state and federal representatives to address core concerns. An informed and vocal majority may be the system's greatest nightmare and the best thing for America.

Value, in health care, is driven by a limited array of factors, including the following:

- *The comparative, true cost of care*—which currently is inaccessible.
- *The comparative clinical quality of care*—for which there is little valid information due to the complexity of evaluating quality. Even so, proxies must be constructed that provide some insight into relative comparative quality between providers.
- *Comparative rates of patient satisfaction with the care they receive*—a measure that Medicare has incorporated into its payment methodology for hospitals. This information is available on the Centers for Medicaid and Medicare Services website.
- *Comparative accessibility of care*—which can be defined as geographic proximity to services, as well as the time intervals between requesting and receiving services (wait times).

Our value equation then looks something like this:

VALUE =   Cost of Care_____

Quality measures + **Patient satisfaction** metrics + **Accessibility**

Bear in mind that even if the information were available to power our value equation, consumers would likely have a difficult time managing key elements of it. The data would need to be translated or processed in a manner that did not dilute its potency yet rendered its essence comprehensible to laypeople.

There still remains one major obstacle to objectifying the value we receive from our hospitals. It is something we've already encountered with physicians: the hospital equivalent of *omertà*.

THE HOSPITALS' CODE OF SILENCE

If hospital executives are truly concerned about the care they deliver to patients, then it would seem logical that they would be forthcoming with information that would help catalyze positive change. But in the world of hospital administration that I've grown accustomed to after three decades, many of my colleagues would consider such thinking to be traitorous.

Hospital leadership teams are not known for their open, enlightened self-examination. Rather, "there is endemic secrecy, deference to authority, defensiveness, and protectionism. Despite much rhetoric about the primacy of patients' interests, it seems that when it matters most, those interests are too often subordinated to the needs and interests of health care organizations and professionals."[49]

How do consumers stand a chance of ever quantifying value in such a culture? Walshe and Shortell are dubious, viewing some health care providers as far more self-serving than patient-focused: "There is a pervasive 'club culture' in which at least some doctors and other health care professionals prioritize their own self-interest above the interests of patients and some health care organization leaders act defensively to protect the institution rather than its patients."[50] Obviously there are exceptions to these broad, sweeping generalizations, but such short-sighted attitudes are, in my experience, far too often the norm.

Only by coming together in groups of sufficient mass to exert market pressure can consumers hope to shatter this barrier to obtaining better, more valued care.

THINGS MAY GET WORSE BEFORE THEY GET BETTER

Hospitals are consolidating at a pace not seen in years. There's safety in numbers, and when the pressure from ratcheted-down reimbursement, complex regulatory requirements, the need for expensive information technology and other factors becomes too much to bear alone, alignment may appear to be an attractive solution for freestanding hospitals, as well as systems.[51]

This trend is affecting both for-profit and not-for-profit providers across many states. Most hospitals involved in such transactions state that their objective is to achieve higher levels of efficiency through initiatives like amortizing the cost of back-office services across a more expansive clinical enterprise. What is left unstated is the increased clout such merged entities wield in their markets—particularly when negotiating rates with insurance companies and other payers.

If the market becomes increasingly oligopolistic, then our ability to control costs will become even weaker, as has been seen in the airline industry where market-dominant carriers are able to inflate prices. The Federal Trade Commission (FTC) should be keeping a careful eye on proposed hospital acquisitions and mergers and not allow predatory pricing to be the outcome of these transactions.

WHAT'S THE MATTER WITH HOSPITALS?

How did hospitals devolve into such a troubled state? Numerous factors have contributed to their poor performance.

The Missing Culture of Innovation

At the top of my list is *the lack of innovation* within the industry. Mind you, I'm not speaking of medical technology, which has burgeoned at an unprecedented pace for the last half-century (generating billions for hospitals, doctors, and the manufacturers of the technology). Here I refer to the lack of creative and strategic thinking that would address the profound deficiencies in today's health care system. Harvard Business School professor Clay Christenson coined a term for what I believe is missing in health care—*disruptive innovation*, which refers to changes that are not merely iterative but that fundamentally restructure the way we do business.

Where are the disruptive innovators in health care? Certainly not running most of today's hospitals. Conservative boards of directors would not allow it, nor would innovators be drawn to the anachronistic world of health care. Unless we want to continue to exist in a health care world akin to the geocentric universe before Galileo, we must invite such disruptive innovators into our midst and brace for the culture shock that, with luck, will follow.

A few health care leaders are strong and confident enough to invite in such catalysts for change. When Rich Hastings, CEO from Saint Luke's Health, invited me into Saint Luke's Health System, he wanted to be intellectually provoked . . . to hear discordant ideas. Under Rich's leadership, the system had grown from one hospital to ten. Part of his success was attributable to the value he placed on out-of-the-box thinking. He welcomed leaders who would shake up the organization and perhaps move it in new directions. That open-minded spirit remained while Rich was at the helm.[52]

Another highly innovative leader with whom I had the pleasure of working is Marvin Pember, the former executive vice president at Indiana University Health (IUH). Marvin helped IUH expand into a major regional provider of care that constantly tested new models for enhancing care delivery.

These gentlemen were worth a great deal to their organizations and the industry because they helped impel it forward.

Overpaying for CEOs Who Function as Custodial Managers

If the majority of senior executives managed like Hastings and Pember, hospitals would likely be far more functional. Yet despite their shortcomings, the majority of hospital and health system CEOs enjoy significant compensation, regardless of whether they work in a not-for-profit or for-profit hospital. This compensation contributes meaningfully to the overall cost of care. It is factored into the charge master as part of the hospital or system's operating costs, which are then amortized against every unit of service, down to the aspirin.

Beyond contributing to escalating costs, there is an ethical issue associated with not-for-profit organizations paying exorbitant salaries to their executives at the same time that they are pleading with the community to contribute to their foundations. Do these contributions enhance care—or the wealth of a privileged few?

> We discovered that some children's hospital CEOs now make over $5 million per year and some had perks including cars, first-class travel, country-club membership, and special retirement packages worth millions.[53]

Adult, acute-care hospitals operate in a similar fashion, with CEOs earning upward of $6 million per year. There are exceptions, however. The CEO of Mayo Clinic, a true thought leader in the industry, earns approximately $2 million annually— one-third as much as some of his colleagues.

When challenged on the appropriateness of high executive compensation, these hospitals often argue that their leaders should be paid at a rate commensurate with what they could command in private industry. I would argue that health care is a calling and that modesty and humility are virtues that not-for-profit health care organizations need to reembrace and reflect in their leader's compensation. Furthermore, I believe that many of today's hospital leaders would struggle in entrepreneurial, market-driven industries.

CEOs are not the only ones drawing big salaries in today's hospitals. Hospitals have rushed to employ physicians at an unprecedented rate in recent years—raising profound issues about their changing role in the health care-delivery system.

The Great Sellout

For many decades, hospitals served as a distribution point for physicians' services. With the exception of selective hospital-based services, such as radiology or emergency, hospitals catered to the needs of their medical staff. It was a symbiotic relationship, but one in which the physician was superordinate.

As physicians increasingly fell prey to diminishing reimbursement and increasing costs, they sought methods for preserving their lifestyle while also extricating themselves from the burden of practice management. Older physicians wanted to ease into retirement without many of the threats that exist in an increasingly hostile health care environment. Younger physicians appeared to be less entrepreneurial than those of preceding generations and more intent on creating effective life-work balance.

Doctors were not the only group subject to these metamorphic pressures. Hospitals were undergoing similar strains. Hospitals also faced another specter—increased competition. Hospital leaders realized that by selectively employing the "right" physicians they could lock in business and stave off competitive threats. They could also command more clout at the bargaining table with insurers.

What began with the employment of primary care physicians soon spread to specialists.

This alignment of needs between two groups that had historically coexisted despite being mutually contemptuous led to a sea change in their relationships. Physicians were willing to sacrifice their independence and control and become workers within the health care system. "Some hospitals are buying physicians' practices outright; 54 percent of physician practices were owned by hospitals in 2012, according to a McKinsey survey, up from 22 percent ten years before."[54]

Why do we care about physician employment if it benefits the hospital and doctors? For some very good reasons:

- It further signals the inevitable progression of our health system from one driven by the need to care for its patients to one driven by profits and business motives. Physicians who were once the overseers of this system and protectors of its core values become pawns within the system—leveraged to the ultimate benefit of the bottom line.
- Employed physicians are under pressure to produce. Previous attempts at physician employment by hospitals in the 1990s resulted in catastrophic losses at some hospitals when physicians, who were guaranteed a salary, simply worked less. New models of employment are now tied to productivity standards, which can incentivize churning of patients. "One doctor I know received an e-mail from his department head that read: 'As we approach the end of the fiscal year, try to do more operations. Your productivity will be used to determine your bonus.'"[55]
- Employed physicians may be pressured to limit referrals only to other physicians employed within their system. Such referral decisions need to be predicated on objective information, not coerced because of obligation through employment.
- By employing physicians, hospitals and health systems gain more clout when negotiating rates, which is at the expense of the payer and ultimately the patient.
- Because physician employment increases the competitive viability of some facilities, it impairs the ability of others. As such, it accel-

erates consolidation within the market—reducing the number of hospital options available to consumers over time.

• As consolidation occurs, hospitals can charge even more.

Conversely, one could argue that physician employment may aid hospitals' efforts at process standardization by assuring physician representation on process-reengineering teams. Such representation, I would argue, could be achieved in a manner other than through employment.

We cannot easily turn back the clock on physician employment, but we can acknowledge the tremendous cost that may ultimately come thanks to this trend. We can also mourn the loss of independence among the former stewards of the industry.

THE ILLUSION OF A MARKET-DRIVEN HEALTH CARE SYSTEM AND THE PROFOUND FEAR OF ANYTHING RESEMBLING "SOCIALIZED MEDICINE"

We have been propagandized to believe that health care is a market-driven industry and, as such, will course correct to meet the demands of the marketplace. As part of our collective brainwashing, we've also been led to believe that any significant changes to the current system may move us closer to socialized medicine, which has been highly demonized.

I was once a passionate advocate for market-driven health care. I believed that, if empowered with the information necessary to make astute purchase decisions, consumers would begin to exert a powerful influence on our health care system. So convinced was I that I agreed to debate a formidable adversary advocating for a single-payer system—a senior editor at *Consumer Reports*. My palms were sweating profusely as I sat backstage at the debate, awaiting my introduction. In front of the curtain sat several hundred people eager to hear a debate on health care reform. Thanks to the Clintons, the topic was on everyone's mind, and the rhetoric regarding proposed solutions was escalating on a daily basis. What no one debated was that our system was desperately ill and unsustainably expensive.

My opponent seemed calm to a fault. She had vociferously argued her position before—that America needed a single-payer system and that market-driven reform was a fantasy. She was smart, articulate, and impeccably well prepared.

When the curtain went up, the fireworks began with me labeling my opponent's cause a cry for socialist medicine in a country built on market-driven dynamics. I insisted that, given time, the market would address the deficiencies in our system without draconian governmental intervention.

A good debate should be won or lost based on the strength of one's logical argument. If I "won" that night, which the audience's reaction seemed to suggest, it was not because of my logic but, rather, my use of rhetoric and propaganda. I did not attack the argument with the intensity that I attacked my opponent.

The debate that night had been sponsored by a Catholic health care system concerned about the changes occurring within the industry. The sisters who had invited me to speak had devoted their lives to providing compassionate care to those in need. Ironically, that night they were handing me a check for an honorarium earned by espousing values that were undoubtedly antithetical to their mission. It was a sobering realization. Before leaving, I handed them back the check and asked that it be put toward a worthy cause.

Twenty years later, I realize that the core premise of my argument—that health care is market-driven—was hopelessly flawed. As I have attempted to demonstrate throughout this book, health care is an aberration in the American marketplace. It is not driven by quality or by value. Therefore, competition among hospitals is more likely to be predicated on propaganda than on any verifiable differences in the value they deliver.

Hospitals and health systems spend millions of dollars on such propaganda designed to achieve two objectives: (1) improve their competitive position in the marketplace and (2) feed the insatiable narcissistic needs of some physicians and board members. In the process, the consumer is bombarded with message after message proclaiming the superiority of one hospital over another. The dollars being spent today on marketing could go a long way toward helping develop and implement transformational strategies for improving the value delivered by our hospitals.

So I guess that makes me a "recovering" health care marketer. *Amazing grace, how sweet the sound / that saved a wretch like me / I once was lost but now I'm found / was blind but now I see.*

WHAT YOU CAN DO TO PROTECT YOUR HEALTH

The best thing you can do to protect your health (and wealth) is stay out of the hospital! I say this only half facetiously. When a hospital represents the most appropriate option for your care, there are a great many things you can do to optimize your chances of an acceptable outcome.

First, understand your physicians' preferences for local hospitals and their reasoning behind such preferences. Second, independently conduct your own due diligence on the local hospital community. It is important that you begin this research before you need hospital services rather than waiting for a crisis. Your proactive research will provide a foundation for making informed decisions. Later, when you have a specific medical need, you can drill deeper into the unique attributes of a given facility.

Base your learning on reliable resources—starting with data provided by CMS. Become familiar with their criteria for evaluating hospitals. Though the terminology may initially be off-putting, stick with it. Your perseverance will pay rewards.

Don't completely discount the propaganda contained on hospitals' websites. There are certainly grains of truth amid the hyperbole. Your job is to separate the two. Statements that make bold claims or boasts may be mere puffery. Assertions supported by hard data, on the other hand, are far more likely to be credible.

Conduct an Internet search for articles that have appeared about your hospital of choice. If you simply type in the name, you will be besieged with hits—including ones that pertain to hospitals with comparable names in other markets. So be creative with your searches. Here are some examples of general and specific queries (executed using Google):

- Chicago hospitals and best mortality rates (19,500,000 hits)
- Chicago hospitals and lowest infection rates (4,210,000 hits)
- Minneapolis hospitals and medical errors (714,000 hits)

- Kansas City hospitals and stereotactic radiosurgery (196,000 hits)
- Cleveland hospitals and aortic valve replacement (97,200 results)

You are not going to weave your way through twenty million references, but even exploring a few dozen may prove to be remarkably enlightening. Furthermore, it should help refine your search criteria so that you get closer and closer to useful information. Be sure to avoid paid advertisements that may appear at the top or the side of your search results.

It is also important to collect anecdotal information from friends, neighbors, and others who have experience with the hospital. Consider the source, and weigh their comments appropriately. A neighbor who happens to be a highly respected cardiac surgeon covering two different health systems may have different insights and biases than a friend from the book club.

With a modicum of effort you should now have the grist you need to create a short list of desired hospitals when the time comes that you need one.

Understand What You Are In For

Before actually utilizing hospital services, more due diligence is called for. The first step is one that we've already discussed—ensuring that you understand your diagnostic or treatment options and that you are in agreement with your physician(s). There should be a shared understanding between you and your proceduralist or surgeon regarding

- what is to be done and the desired outcome;
- the manner in which it will be done;
- the ramifications of the surgery and potential adverse consequences or risks;
- the time required for surgery;
- who will perform the surgery (will residents be involved, for instance);
- the anticipated recovery time;
- the potential need for subsequent surgeries;
- anesthesia coverage; and

- scheduling the procedure. If you are having a procedure requiring an inpatient stay, request that it not be performed on a Friday. If at all possible, you want to avoid spending time in the hospital during any part of the weekend, when staffing shrinks noticeably and key services may be unavailable.

Regardless of whether you are about to receive hospital-based inpatient or outpatient services, there are certain things you should seek to understand, including

- the volume of comparable procedures performed at the hospital and by the physician;
- some indication of outcomes, though this data is not easy to obtain;
- information about adverse events that occur in the hospital relative to its peers;
- information about patient satisfaction with the hospital relative to its peers;
- proximity of the hospital to you and your loved one (and advocate);
- the type of hospital . . . and the importance of these characteristics to you (e.g., do you wish to be treated in an academic versus community hospital, or faith-based versus for-profit, or specialty versus general acute care); and
- staffing ratios (and the RN ratio).

Increasing the Odds of Surviving and Thriving

Now that you have done your due diligence and settled on a facility and provider, you need to increase the probability of a good outcome. There are several things that you can do to optimize a successful encounter with the hospital:

- When going to the hospital or outpatient facility, it is essential that you be accompanied by a family member or trusted friend who can act as your ombudsman for the duration of your encounter. This person should serve as both an advocate for your rights as well as an extra set of eyes and ears that monitors, questions, and records all the care you receive. They should not bat an eye at asking for an explanation from any care procedures.

- Just as we were once advised to not buy cars manufactured on Friday because they were more prone to defects, you should avoid scheduling surgeries on Friday or the weekend for much the same reason. In fact, according to *Consumer Reports*, your chances of dying from surgery increase late in the week and over the weekend—a time when hospital staffing often changes.

- Avoid acquiring a hospital-induced injury or infection by following directions regarding your personal hygiene, collaborating with attempts to get you on your feet so that you avoid dangerous blood clots, and providing the hospital with a complete list of your medications in order to avoid negative synergistic interactions with drugs that may be prescribed while you are an inpatient.

Price Should Matter to You

Don't hesitate to ask about the costs associated with your potential hospitalization—assuming that your condition is not emergent and permits such discernment. Though hospital staff may stammer and stutter when asked for the price of an upcoming procedure, remain resolute in your need for the information.

Be sure to provide all your insurance information and verify that the price being quoted properly reflects all network discounts you are due. Also ask what is not included in the price (e.g., the surgeon's fees and anesthesiologist's fees).

Once you obtain the information, assuming it is somewhat accurate, you need to put it in context relative to other providers in your market. The problem is coming up with comparative price data from other providers. There are emerging Internet-based resources that claim to give you a leg up when seeking to make such comparisons. One such resource is the Healthcare Bluebook.[56]

Healthcare Bluebook was founded by Jeff Rice, MD, a self-proclaimed entrepreneur who did his medical training at Duke University. He stayed on to become the director of Managed Care at Duke, where he was responsible for thirty thousand insured lives. His professional experience led him to conclude that not only was there tremendous price variation across providers but that patients were generally quite oblivious to it.[57]

Healthcare Bluebook is designed to help patients, employers, and payers understand what "fair pricing" is for a procedure in their community. Rice stated that, at his organization, "we find that fair pricing is usually between the thirty-third and fifty-fifth percentile. Our data comes from our employer and payer clients. It is very robust and extremely accurate."[58]

Dr. Rice shared with me data related to colonoscopy prices in one market. Prices varied from $900 to $3,500, which he indicated is relatively typical for many services across most markets. Dr. Rice said that the greatest determinant of price was the location of service—with academic medical centers being the most expensive and physician-owned facilities being the least.[59]

Rice's message is simple: "You should be able to find a local, in-network provider willing to provide the service at or below our fair price." He claims that his site has fair pricing for 90 percent of the top procedures by volume. When I asked about cancer treatments, such as radiation therapy for prostate, Dr. Rice indicated that the site does not have information for these types of services.[60]

The bottom line: I wouldn't accept the Healthcare Bluebook's data as the gospel, but I would consider it to be an interesting data point perhaps worthy of consideration.

After your hospital encounter, be certain to methodically check your bill for inaccuracies. Chances are that it contains errors that you could end up paying for. If you need assistance deciphering, checking, or negotiating your bill, there are a growing number of reputable resources to assist you on the Internet by searching "hospital billing assistance" or similar terms.

A Few More Words of Cautionary Advice

- You should have a complete understanding of the procedure and its potential risks as part of the informed-consent process—do not sign anything until you understand exactly what treatment you are consenting to have performed.
- If your insurance company is balking at the proposed procedure or hospitalization, take note—they may be acting in your best interest.

Insurance companies will frequently conduct a "peer-to-peer" review
of a planned treatment when it deviates from accepted standards. If
there is a clear justification for such deviation, the insurance company generally approves it. If not, you may want to get a second opinion
before deciding that your insurer is inhibiting your ability to get the
care you need.

- Before any type of procedure, be certain that the medical team ver-
ifies with you what they are planning to do to what area of the body.
- Be sure that they have marked your body appropriately before surgery.
- Ensure that all caregivers wash their hands before examining you to
prevent a hospital-acquired infection.
- Be cognizant that many hospital injuries take the form of falls—
usually when a patient is navigating the short distance from bed to
bathroom. Ask for help getting up from your hospital bed.
- Be certain that your pain is being adequately and appropriately managed.

Survival Manuals for Hospital Patients

I've barely scratched the surface relative to the steps you and your
advocate must take to optimize your chances of a safe and positive
hospital experience. I strongly recommend you read several books that
will help prepare you for future hospital encounters:

- Though somewhat dated by its original publication in 1985,
Charles Inlander's *Take This Book to the Hospital: A Consumer
Guide to Surviving Your Hospital Stay* is a patient-advocacy classic. It has undergone several updates and is available via Ama-
zon.com.
- *Safe and Sound in the Hospital,* by Karen Curtiss, provides step-
by-step instructions, checklists, and tools to aiding loved ones in
ensuring that they get the care they need and deserve.

There are many more resources a few clicks away on the Internet. A
little time invested before a hospital encounter can make a profound
difference in your care experience.

MYTH 7
"THE PRESCRIPTION I WAS GIVEN IS SAFE, PROVEN, AND EFFECTIVE"

When Matt Miller, a seemingly well-adjusted middle schooler, began showing signs of emotional distress following a recent family move, his parents, Mark and Cheryl, became appropriately concerned. The once engaging and popular thirteen-year-old was becoming withdrawn, and his performance at school was in a precipitous decline.[1]

At first, Matt's parents thought it might simply be a transient period of adjustment to a new school and new friends . . . after all, they had only moved fifteen minutes away from their old home. As Matt's behavior persisted, however, they realized that their son might be in trouble.

With the encouragement of school personnel, "on June 30, 1997, the Millers took Matt to see Dr. Douglas Geenens, a child psychiatrist referred to them by Matt's primary care physician."[2] *Over the course of two appointments, Dr. Geenens diagnosed Matt as suffering from depression and recommended that he take an antidepressant known as Zoloft.*[3]

Dr. Geenens concluded the appointment by addressing questions from the Millers, assuaging their concerns regarding side-effects, and indicated that he would visit with the family again in August.

Their son never made it to his next appointment. Within days of beginning treatment with Zoloft, Matt's behavior seemed to change. The family reported increased restlessness, agitation, and ultimately anger:

> On Sunday night, July 27, at around 11:30, Matt was still on the phone with his girlfriend. Mark went to his son's room to tell him to hang up and go to bed. "I didn't yell at him, but I was firm," Mark recalled. Matt threw the phone down and angrily slammed the door in his father's face, something he'd never done before. Mark went back to his room and asked Cheryl if he should go back in and talk to him. Cheryl thought they ought to wait until the morning. "He's finally just getting settled," she told Mark. "We don't want to rile him up again." When Cheryl went in to awaken Matt the following morning, she found him hanging by a belt from a laundry hook in his closet. [4]

There is nothing more horrific to a parent than finding their child dead from suicide. The Millers' grief was overwhelming. Thanks to an outpouring of sympathy and care, coupled with a resolute sense of faith, Mark and Cheryl somehow managed through their darkest days.

After two years of contemplation, they decided to file a lawsuit against Pfizer, the manufacturer of Zoloft. As the case moved forward, they discovered how equivocal the evidence could be. Experts argued whether Zoloft and other chemically similar compounds (SSRIs) played a key role in exacerbating dangerous and aberrant behavior. In the end, the Millers were unsuccessful in prosecuting their claim.

There was one small victory, however. The FDA validated a potential correlation between adolescent use of antidepressants and the development of suicidal thinking. "Now all antidepressants, including SSRIs like Prozac, Zoloft, Paxil, Lexapro, Luvox, and Celexa, must carry a black-box warning label, the regulatory agency's strongest kind, making a possible suicide link explicit and all but ensuring a significant decrease in their use among young people."[5] Nothing would bring Matt back, but at least other parents might be spared the tragedy they had endured.

My stepson, Tim, is the same age that Matt would be if he were alive today. In fact, Tim and Matt were friends, living but blocks apart and attending the same grade school. I can't imagine losing Tim or any of our children. Hence, it's almost incomprehensible to me that a corporation would knowingly put profits ahead of a child's well-being; yet numerous parents have made that allegation against a cadre of pharmaceutical giants who manufacture antidepressants and other potent medications. In the case of the Millers, the jury found in favor of the corporation. In other cases, faced with other manufacturers, juries have found in favor of the plaintiff.

Better life through medicine—that's what we have been promised. Whether it's the "purple pill" or a powerful antidepressant, we can't imagine life without our drugs. Selective serotonin-reuptake inhibitors (SSRIs), such as the one taken by Matt, often top the list of most-frequently prescribed drugs in America, leading one to believe in their inherent safety and effectiveness.

Yet these and other drugs come at a price—both literally and figuratively. They account for billions of dollars in profits, and they have the potential to harm untold millions of patients who remain blissfully unaware of their hidden dangers. For us to understand how such drugs could enter the market, we must first understand a bit about pharmaceutical research.

LIES, DAMN LIES, AND STATISTICS

It's America—where everyone is allowed to make a profit for an honest day's work. So why pick on the pharmaceutical companies? Well, what if that work is not so honest? What if the public, even the medical profession, has been duped through the manipulation of research to support questionable drugs? Is that okay? And what if people die as a result? Is that simply the cost of doing business for the nation's most profitable industry?

There's a growing body of evidence to suggest the gross manipulation of research used to support the approval and subsequent sales of drugs. This manipulation includes both the outright falsification of data and the suppression of key research findings—leading to the misinterpretation of a drug's efficacy or safety. Rather than being rare events, some of these practices appear to be standard operating procedure within the industry.

This bastardization of the research process is occurring concurrently with a shift in how research is conducted. Pharmaceutical research has long been the bastion of major academic organizations, the majority of which have well-established reputations to protect. As such, every research study must be approved by an internal review board that scrutinizes the research design to ensure it is ethical and appropriate.

In an effort to exert greater control over the research process, pharmaceutical companies have moved much of their business from the hallowed halls of academia to for-profit, contract-research organizations (CROs). CRO-driven studies are referred to as *industry sponsored*.

There is a pervasive problem with CROs, according to author Ben Goldacre, MD, and the manner in which they come to conclusions that are highly beneficial to their sponsor. "Industry-sponsored trials give favorable results," says Goldacre, "and that is not my opinion or a hunch from the occasional passing study. This is a very well-documented problem, and it has been researched extensively, without anybody stepping out to take effective action."[6]

It is not a matter of simply tipping the scale a bit in favor of pharma. Some of the practices engaged in by CROs are downright fraudulent. Garver et al. provided a glimpse into the most egregious of these practices in a series of articles appearing in *Scientific American* and on the ProPublica website.[7]

The first article focused on problems with a well-established contract-research organization known as Cetero, which served pharmaceutical manufacturers across the globe. When three FDA agents showed up on his doorstep one May morning in 2010, Cetero CEO Chinna Pamidi seemed largely unfazed. In a conversation with lead agent Patrick Stone, Pamidi confessed to the fraudulent nature of his company's research.[8]

Just how bad was the deception? "The FDA eventually concluded that the lab's violations were so 'egregious' and pervasive that studies conducted there between April 2005 and August 2009 might be worthless."[9] This research did not affect merely one or two drugs. "About one hundred drugs, including sophisticated chemotherapy compounds and addictive prescription painkillers, had been approved for sale in the United States at least in part on the strength of Cetero Houston's tainted tests."[10]

What is equally alarming is the manner in which the FDA managed their discovery. According to Garver, rather than go public with this astonishing and disheartening finding, "the agency decided to handle the matter quietly, evaluating the medicines with virtually no public disclosure of what it had discovered. It pulled none of the drugs from the market."[11]

Cetero is not the only bad apple among CROs. Garver and his colleagues also called attention to trouble at MDS Pharma Services:

- The first hint of trouble at MDS Pharma came in July 2003, when FDA investigators found problems with a study of a generic form of the allergy medicine Claritin during an inspection of MDS Pharma's facility in St. Laurent, Quebec.[12]
- In another inspection, lasting more than three weeks in September and October 2004, FDA investigators found multiple problems with MDS studies.[13]
- In January 2007, three and a half years after first finding problems at MDS, the FDA informed drug makers that studies done by MDS between 2000 and 2004 needed to be reevaluated. FDA officials told the media that 217 generic drugs were potentially implicated, 140 of which had already been approved for sale.[14]
- The FDA made no effort to warn doctors or patients that now had doubts about the data underlying some of the drugs it had approved.[15]

Less egregious but far more rampant are the numerous practices that distort research findings. Chief among them is the practice of publishing only those studies that support the efficacy and safety of a drug so that physicians and their patients receive a highly biased view of the results of clinical trials: "Sometimes drug companies conduct lots of trials, and when they see that the results are unflattering, they simply fail to publish them."[16]

A case in point is the research to support the efficacy, safety, and sales of the most widely prescribed antidepressants. Most of these drugs belong to a category known as *SSRIs*—selective serotonin-reuptake inhibitors—referring to their mechanism of action within the brain. This class of drug and its close cousins account for billions in pharmaceutical sales . . . but do they work as promised?

In 2008 a group of researchers decided to check for publication of every trial that had ever been reported to the US Food and Drug Administration for all the antidepressants that came onto the market between 1987 and 2004. The researchers found seventy-four studies in total, representing 12,500 patients' worth of data. Thirty-eight of these trials had positive results and found that the new drug worked;

thirty-six were negative. Thirty-seven of the positive trials—all but one—were published in full, often with much fanfare. But the trials with negative results had a very different fate: only three were published. Twenty-two were simply lost to history. . . . The remaining eleven [that] had negative results in the FDA summaries did appear in the academic literature but were written up as if the drug was a success.[17]

Physicians, who rely on seemingly objective, peer-reviewed studies to make informed decisions on their patients' behalf, are relying on half-truths. The above-mentioned 2008 study "very clearly exposed a broken system: in reality we have thirty-eight positive trials and thirty-seven negative ones; in the academic literature we have forty-eight positive trials and three negative ones."[18]

If you examine the research supporting individual drugs, the picture of deception remains equally disheartening. A case in point is reboxetine—an SNRI (selective norepinephrine-reuptake inhibitor) used to treat depression, panic attacks, and related conditions. Goldacre shares a provocative study in which all the research supporting the use of this drug was analyzed:

In October 2010 a group of researchers [was] finally able to bring together all the trials that had ever been conducted on reboxetine. When all of this trial data was put together it produced a shocking picture. Seven trials had been conducted comparing reboxetine against placebo. Only one, conducted in 254 patients, had a neat, positive result, and that one was published in an academic journal, for doctors and researchers to read. But six more trials were conducted, in almost ten times as many patients. All of them showed that reboxetine was no better than a dummy sugar pill. None of these trials was published.[19]

Goldacre's conclusion was simple and powerful: "In the published data, reboxetine was a safe and effective drug. In reality, it was no better than a sugar pill, and, worse, it does more harm than good."[20]

It's not just the antidepressant research that is suspect. Goldacre found that "in 2006 researchers looked into every trial of psychiatric drugs in four academic journals over a ten-year period, finding 542 trial outcomes in total. Industry sponsors got favorable outcomes for their own drug 78 percent of the time, while independently funded trials only gave a positive result in 48 percent of cases."[21] Some research psychiatrists argue that such findings are not an invalidation of the efficacy of the drugs but, rather, spotlight deficiencies in research methodologies, including poor selection criteria for inclusion in the studies.

These misrepresentations appear to follow the money—the greater the potential sales and profits associated with a drug, the more tempting it appears to be to suppress information. Such is the case with one of the most commonly prescribed "blockbuster" drugs—the statins. Statins are used to reduce serum cholesterol levels. When first brought to market, they were heralded as safe yet potent life savers that would help keep cardiovascular disease at bay.

A cardiologist once said to me, "I think everyone over the age of thirty-five should be on a statin; there's little harm and a great deal of good that would come of it." However, meta-analysis of the research literature seems to suggest otherwise. Nortin Hadler, MD, professor of Medicine and Microbiology/Immunology at the University of North Carolina, asserts that "there are serious questions whether statin treatment affords any meaningful advantage to people who have not had a heart attack."[22]

Hadler's bold assertion regarding a mainstay of modern medicine gains support when one examines the lack of impartiality associated with the research. Goldacre found that "in 2007 researchers looked at every published trial that set out to explore the benefit of a statin. This study found 192 trials in total, either comparing one statin against another or comparing a statin against a different kind of treatment. Once the researchers controlled for other factors, they found that industry-funded trials were twenty times more likely to give results favoring the test drug."[23] How do pharma and its coconspirators, the CROs, con sophisticated audiences such as physicians? It sometimes begins with the research design or patient selection—both of which can lead to artificially positive results for the drug. Next, a research study may be stopped midstream if it is failing to yield the desired positive outcome or is showing a negative outcome for the drug being tested. For those studies not stopped in time to prevent the airing of negative results, the findings may be quickly buried.

Any student of statistics knows that data can be manipulated in many ways to misrepresent the truth. Hence, the old saying "There are lies, damn lies, and statistics." A negative result may be masked behind a statistical facade that makes it look positive. The result is a much-distorted picture of the true efficacy and safety of innumerable drugs or classes of drugs on the market.

Research outcomes are often fed to the media as percentages, leading to bold headlines. It's not uncommon to see or hear about a new drug that appears to reduce mortality for a given condition by 50 percent. What's not included in the sound bite are the actual numbers. In a given trial, that may mean that only one person in ten thousand died from a condition versus the expected two. A headline declaring that "Drug Z Reduces Death Rate by 1 in 10,000" would likely not garner much attention.

Remember, your physician is often relying on the data provided by the pharmaceutical industry and its collaborators . . . including the professional medical associations to which your physician belongs. Yet even here there appears to be complicity: "Fries and Krishnan studied all the research abstracts presented at the 2001 American College of Rheumatology meetings [that] reported any kind of trial, and acknowledged industry sponsorship, in order to find out what proportion had results that favored the sponsor's drug. The results from every RCT (forty-five out of forty-five) favored the drug of the sponsor."[24]

When it comes to the research supporting pharmaceuticals, it would appear that the only thing we can absolutely rely on is the profound lack of truth and integrity behind the research. As Goldacre warns us, "because researchers are free to bury any result they please, patients are exposed to harm on a staggering scale throughout the whole of medicine, from research to practice. Doctors can have no idea about the true effects of the treatments they give. Does this drug really work best, or have I simply been deprived of half the data?"[25]

Though not directing his comments specifically at pharmaceutical researchers, Anthony L. Zietman, MD, editor-in-chief of the *International Journal of Radiation Oncology*, offered these sobering thoughts relative to the state of today's research:

> One of the greatest, and sadly all-too-common, challenges facing contemporary medical-journal editors is the adjudication of ethical-integrity issues. I had originally presumed that this would be just an occasional role, but it transpires that these problems are quite wide-

spread, ranging from unconscious and unwitting naïveté to the conscious and willful betrayal of scientific trust.

Between 2001 and 2010, the number of manuscripts accepted by listed medical journals increased by 44 percent. The number of retracted papers over the same period, however, went up nineteenfold! It has been estimated that the majority of the retractions resulted from conscious misdemeanors rather than honest errors.[26]

If you are wondering why an industry would go to such lengths to bastardize research findings and deceive not only the public but physicians as well, you need look no further than the bottom line of major pharmaceutical manufacturers.

THE PILL BUSINESS

The most profitable business in America is peddling drugs. Pharmaceutical companies enjoy profit margins that are the envy of every other industry in America, despite the industry's protestations regarding the burdensome costs of bringing new drugs to market. "In 2002, for example, the top ten drug companies in the United States had a median profit margin of 17 percent, compared with only 3.1 percent for all the other industries on the Fortune 500 list. Indeed, subtracting losses from gains, those ten companies made more in profits that year than the other 490 companies put together."[27]

The year 2002 was not an aberration. Like an annuity, the drug companies have continued to return consistently strong returns year after year. In an August 2009 article in *U.S. News & World Report*, author Rick Newman relied on data from Capital IQ to examine the profitability of the nation's largest health care companies. Though the list included major insurers, device manufacturers, and hospital companies, the top six performers by profit-margin percentage were all pharmaceuticals/biotechnology manufacturers. Coming in seventh was UnitedHealth, the nation's largest health insurance provider. It earned a paltry 4.1 percent—or less than one-seventh of the profit margin (by percentage) enjoyed by Amgen:

- Gilead Sciences (biotechnology): 37.6 percent profit margin
- Amgen (biotechnology): 30.6 percent

- Johnson & Johnson (drug manufacturer): 20.8 percent
- GlaxoSmithKline (drug manufacturer): 17.4 percent
- Pfizer (drug manufacturer): 16.3 percent
- Celgene Corp. (biotechnology): 11.9 percent
- UnitedHealth Group (health care plans): 4.1 percent[28]

Newman concludes that "some of these numbers are sure to be off-putting to Americans who are making sacrifices to pay for health care or can't afford it at all. Yet industries like pharma and biotech remain strong job creators that have held up well during the recession, and they represent parts of the global economy where America still enjoys a leading position."[29]

Mr. Newman may be able to see the silver lining in the outrageous profits enjoyed by pharma, but not me. Instead, I think about the people in our society who have to choose between putting food on the table or paying for their medications. Then I think about 20 percent and greater profit margins and wonder what has happened to our values.

Social injustice aside, there's also the issue of the value delivered by these drugs. "The major drug manufacturers have a 23 percent profit margin . . . and this is all happening despite the fact that researchers are having a very difficult time showing that there's much benefit—either in longevity or quality of life—to all these new and incredibly expensive treatments."[30]

WHAT WE SPEND ON DRUGS

As should be obvious by now, Americans have developed an expensive habit. In 2011 we spent more than $265 billion on retail prescriptions. Though spending appears to be moderating due to increased use of generics and other factors, our bill is nonetheless expected to exceed $280 billion in 2013.

With the pace of sales slowing, consulting giant McKinsey Global Institute sounded a warning for the pharmaceutical industry:

> The good old days of the pharmaceutical industry are gone forever. Even an improved global economic climate is unlikely to halt efforts by the developed world's governments to contain spending on drugs. Emerging markets will follow their lead and pursue further spend-

ing-control measures. Regulatory requirements—particularly the linkage among the benefits, risks, and cost of products—will increase, while the industry pipeline shows little sign of delivering sufficient innovation to compensate for such pressures. These factors suggest that the industry is heading toward a world where its profit margins will be substantially lower than they are today. This dramatic situation requires Big Pharma executives to envision responses that go well beyond simply tinkering with the cost base or falling back on mergers and acquisitions.[31]

But as McKinsey consultants know all too well, the pharmaceutical industry is far too aggressive to sit back and watch our national drug tab dwindle. As generics replace once-expensive "blockbuster" drugs, major pharmaceutical manufacturers are implementing a new strategy that promises alleged benefits to patients while guaranteeing ongoing returns to shareholders.

PERSONALIZED MEDICINE: THE KEY TO PRESERVING PHARMACEUTICAL PROFITS

Just as medical technology has advanced from the simple X-ray to MRIs, CTs, and PET scans, pharmaceuticals have advanced from arsenic-based compounds and radium salts to targeted molecular therapies. Today's pharmaceuticals are capable of addressing a broad array of maladies. Tomorrow's drugs, if true to promise, will be the silver bullets of medicine, tapping into our unique genetic profiles to stop the ravaging effects of diseases like cancer.

No one could be more eager to embrace this new paradigm than pharmaceutical executives. As such, the drug companies have been migrating their business from a model predicated on one-size-fits-all blockbuster drugs to highly personalized, immensely expensive therapies.

Kate Thomas called attention to this strategic shift in the March 18, 2013, issue of the *New York Times*, noting that "some are warning that the ever-expanding use of generics has masked a growing problem for the government, insurers, and others who pay the bill for prescription drugs: the rising cost of complex specialty medicines that treat cancer, rheumatoid arthritis, and other diseases."[32] Many of these drugs cost upward of $10,000 per month—costs that are not merely unfathomable but arguably unsustainable. Try telling that to a dying cancer patient who may eke out an additional six months of life thanks to a medication.

How much money do pharmaceutical manufacturers stand to make on drugs like these? If history is any indication of future profitability, the bounty will be immense.

Some pharmaceutical/biotechnology companies have gone so far as to seek patent protection for specific human genes. Myriad Diagnostics, the company responsible for identifying the BRAC1 and 2 genes, is a prime example. The BRAC1 mutation in women predisposes them to a 50 to 80 percent likelihood of developing breast cancer, as well as a 25 to 50 percent chance of developing ovarian cancer at some point during their lives.

Myriad sought to protect its diagnostic discovery by patenting its research—thus preventing other companies from offering BRAC testing. In June 2013 the U.S. Supreme Court ruled that Myriad could not prevent other companies from competing: "Genes and the information they encode are not patent eligible under §101 simply because they have been isolated from the surrounding genetic material."[33] There are already signs that this decision will introduce a new order of competition, thus reducing the cost of BRAC testing.

INCREASING OUR APPETITE THROUGH MARKETING

Drugs should "sell themselves" based on proven efficacy and safety. Physicians will embrace compounds for which the scientific evidence supports the use of the drug within a given clinical context. However, when the evidence is nonexistent, tampered with, or equivocal, marketing steps in to the rescue.

A case in point is antidepressants, where we've seen a substantial level of controversy surrounding the purported efficacy of the drugs. Perhaps that's why in "2010 spending to promote Cymbalta, an antidepressant, equaled $620 million—or 19.4 percent of total drug sales. Lexapro, another antidepressant, was not far behind with total marketing expenditures of $400 million or 14.3 percent of sales."[34]

When one looks across the industry, rather than focusing on each drug, the numbers spent on marketing grow exponentially. A 2007 article by McFadden et al. stated that "marketing costs exceed 30 percent of revenues for the pharmaceutical industry, with over 90 percent of the effort aimed at physicians."[35] That translated into $28 billion spent on pharmaceutical promotion to consumers and providers in 2010.[36] Of the total dollars spent in 2010, $23 billion went to promotion to providers, or approximately 80 percent.[37]

Whether 80 percent or 90, the vast majority of pharma's marketing dollars focus on the person with greatest influence on drug sales—the physician. Physician marketing takes many forms—from bringing lunches to physicians' offices to sponsoring "educational" conferences. The largest expense, however, is associated with free samples of drugs left by detailers.[38]

One of the most controversial forms of marketing is the provision of gifts to physicians. Those gifts range from trinkets to checks for hundreds of thousands of dollars: "The main objective of drug-company giving is to create relationships and interest on the part of the recipient physicians that conflict with their primary obligation to act in the best interest of their patients."[39]

DOCTORS ON THE TAKE

Though not technically gifts, other questionable practices within the industry involve payments made by pharma (and device manufacturers) to physicians in support of the drugs or devices they produce. These payments are in no way trivial: A *New York Times* article appearing on May 13, 2013, told the story of Dr. Alfred J. Tria, chief of orthopedics at a major teaching hospital in New Brunswick, New Jersey. "In 2010, Dr. Tria earned $421,905 from private industry—more than any other Massachusetts-licensed physician that year."[40]

An increasing number of studies are examining these payments and the potential conflicts of interest that they engender. Once such study looked at payments to physicians and researchers within the state of Texas. It found that "from 2009 to early 2011, at least twenty-five thousand Texas physicians and researchers received a combined $57 million—and probably far more—in cash payments, research money, free meals, travel, and other perks, according to data culled from twelve drug companies and provided by the nonprofit investigative news organization ProPublica. Dozens of these medical professionals were paid more than $100,000 each during the period."[41]

A similar study examined payments to doctors in Massachusetts: "Gifts and payments to physicians from drug and medical-device companies have been rampant in medicine for decades. Over a two-and-a-half-year period, device and drug companies shelled out over $76 million just to physicians licensed in Massachusetts, according to a study published online this month in the *New England Journal of Medicine*. That amount does not include outlays of less than $50, which are exempt from disclosure."[42]

The pharmaceutical companies begin peddling their influence at the earliest point in emerging physicians' careers—while they are still in medical school. Pauline Chen, MD, recounts her medical school experience with drug reps in a provocative article appearing in the *New York Times*:

> As trainees in a large teaching hospital, we knew numerous sales reps by name and the products they peddled; and it was odd, even disappointing, to go to an educational conference where one of them was not standing next to a table laden with tchotchkes, information brochures, and free takeout.
>
> In an environment where no one, including senior doctors, ever questioned the presence of sales reps, we didn't think too hard about why they might have been so friendly and helpful as they were. We didn't ask where the money for all these giveaways was coming from, and we were rarely curious about who these reps actually were. (I only ever knew their first names.)[43]

Physicians often argue that these gifts and/or payments pose no conflict of interest because they have no effect on their practice patterns. Such a claim would suggest that these doctors are above human frailty. Physicians may think that they are immune to manipulation by advertising and marketing, but as has been pointed out by Coste and other researchers, "the success of pharmaceutical marketing illustrates that physicians are as susceptible to target marketing as others."[44]

This statement is not mere opinion but is supported by numerous researchers within the industry:

- In a meta-analysis of all major studies conducted to date on the topic, author Ashley Wazana, MD, concluded that "the present extent of physician-industry interactions appears to affect prescribing and professional behavior and should be further addressed at the level of policy and education."[45] Wazana estimated that pharmaceutical-company spending on physicians amounted to anywhere between $8,000 to $13,000 per year per physician.[46]
- Dr. Robert Steinbrook, former deputy editor at the *New England Journal of Medicine*, warned that "these relationships . . . can influence prescribing behavior and the use of medical devices and supplies, increase the cost of care, create a mind-set of entitlement among doctors, and undermine the independence and integrity of the profession."[47]
- Ramshaw and Murphy found that "state records [in Texas] show that of the seventy-four doctors and psychiatrists statewide who have routinely prescribed the highest number of costly antipsychotic drugs to patients on Medicaid . . . ten received payments from drug companies in 2009–2011 from $11,000 to $180,000 each. All but one got the payments from the maker of the drug they most commonly prescribed."[48]

It is interesting to note that it doesn't take a large gift or payment to have a dramatic impact on a physician. Quite the contrary, "a large body of evidence from the social sciences shows that behavior can be influenced by gifts of negligible value."[49]

Despite the overwhelming data, studies continue to show that most physicians believe that common marketing activities engaged in by industry are appropriate, according to a survey of nearly six hundred physicians associated with the Mount Sinai School of Medicine and its affiliated hospitals: "Participants had overall positive attitudes toward marketing-related interactions with the pharmaceutical or device industries. Most believed it was acceptable to receive gifts and lunches, and few thought that industry representatives should be banned from meeting with physicians."[50]

Two other findings from this study are worthy of mention: (1) "surgeons were more likely overall to rate gifts from industry . . . as appropriate"[51] and (2) "participants believed that other physicians were more likely than they to be influenced by industry marketing (284 [52.2 percent] vs. 194 [35.6 percent]).”[52]

If you are wondering if your physician accepts payments from drug or device manufacturers, you will soon be able to find out. Thanks to the Physician Payments Sunshine Act, this information will be available online in 2014. Though consumers need to be cautioned not to draw erroneous conclusions regarding the appropriateness of these payments to their physicians, they are certainly free to ask questions about the physician's impartiality—particularly when their doctor is recommending the use of a drug or device manufactured by the physician's benefactor.

INFLUENCING THE INFLUENCERS

If influencing individual physicians is powerful, imagine what could be accomplished by exerting influence over the panels of physicians who set the standards for when drugs should be prescribed. When the recommended maximum, unmedicated level of cholesterol drops from 240 to 200, the number of prescriptions rises like a thermometer on a scorching summer day. If you think that such panels are above such malarkey, take a look at the evidence to the contrary:

- “A paper Dr. Korenstein [an associate professor at Mount Sinai] published in 2011 found that more than a dozen expert panels that developed national clinical-practice guidelines for managing diabetes and high cholesterol were dominated by physicians with financial conflicts of interest—that is, they were receiving payment from companies with an interest in how these diseases are managed.”[53]
- “Among the 288 panel members, 138 (48 percent) reported conflicts of interest at the time of the publication of the guidelines and 150 (52 percent) either stated that they had no such conflicts or did not have an opportunity to declare any. Among seventy-three panels who formally declared no conflicts, eight (11 percent) were found to have one or more. Twelve of the fourteen guideline panels evaluated identified chairs, among whom six had financial conflicts of interest. Overall, 150 (52 percent) panel

members had conflicts of which 138 were declared and twelve were undeclared."[54]

- "The prevalence of financial conflicts of interest and their under-reporting by members of panels producing clinical-practice guidelines on hyperlipidemia or diabetes was high, and a relatively high proportion of guidelines did not have public disclosure of conflicts of interest."[55]

SELLING DRUGS ON THE STREET: DIRECT-TO-CONSUMER ADVERTISING

Before the 1990s, virtually all promotion of prescription drugs was targeted to physicians. That changed dramatically in 1997, when the FDA modified its restrictions on consumer advertising. "Spending by the drug industry on [direct-to-consumer] advertising grew from $791 million in 1996 to $3.2 billion in 2003, mostly for promotion of fifty brand-name drugs."[56] Though it decreased between 2006 and 2010, that number had nonetheless grown to $5 billion by 2010.[57]

These are not public-service announcements designed to educate the public. They are the modern equivalent of hucksterism—the broadcast version of a sandwich board proclaiming the power of Baldwin's Herbal Tonic Mixture, *Nature's General Restorer of the System and Purifier of the Blood*. Manufacturers are not imparting objective information; they are generating tremendous increases in sales by capitalizing on the vulnerability and naïveté of the lay public.

Physicians, wishing to keep their patients happy, often acquiesce to their request for a prescription that they've seen advertised on TV. In a study of primary care physicians in Sacramento and Vancouver, BC, "patients who requested DTCA [direct-to-consumer-advertised] drugs were nearly seventeen times as likely to receive one or more new prescriptions as patients who did not request medicines. Nearly nine out of ten such patients received prescriptions for either the drug they had requested or an alternative."[58]

Though the benefits enjoyed by the patient may be minimal, the benefits felt by pharma are immediate: "IMS Health found in its study of 'return on investment' in DTC advertising that at least 90 percent of the brands demonstrated positive returns."[59] This research further determined that every dollar spent on DTC advertising generated an average increase of $4.20 in sales volume. Of the brands directly marketed to consumers, "The best-performing brand yielded a return of $6.50 per dollar invested."[60]

I worked on a DTC marketing campaign for a major pharmaceutical manufacturer a number of years ago. Our goal was to take a drug that effectively treated incontinence and reposition it as also being appropriate for the treatment of urinary frequency, a much more common complaint. By doing so, the size of the hypothetical market for this drug would increase dramatically . . . and it did. My client watched contentedly as sales for this drug soared from $300 million to close to $1 billion in a few years—with no underlying change to the actual drug! A difference of $700 million in sales pays for plenty of DTC advertising.

Why are these promotions so effective? For three primary reasons:

1. Our need to believe that pharmaceuticals can help remove us from the inescapable disease, decline, and death that are part of the human condition.
2. The illusory belief that we know more about the actual efficacy and safety of these drugs than we really do: "Consumer knowledge and confidence in prescription medications is high. Eighty-eight percent of prescription-medication users believe they understand how their meds work. Eighty-seven percent believe they understand the risks and side effect, and 86 percent are confident their medication is effective."[61]
3. Our erroneous conclusion that there are multiple safeguards barring misinformation and dangerous drugs from affecting us—be it the FDA, our personal physician, or the ethics of the pharmaceutical industry.

Some drugs do work as advertised and with minimal risk to the patient. Some drugs appear to work but perhaps based more on the placebo effect than true efficacy. And some drugs are either ineffective or dangerous or both.

GENERATING BUSINESS BY INVENTING DISEASE

The pharmaceutical industry has found another fascinating way to increase sales. It relies on either fabricating new diseases or grossly exaggerating the incidence of such diseases in the population. The manufacturers then recommend their products for the treatment of these real and imagined diseases.

The most recent example of such fabrication is for men "suffering" the effects of low testosterone ("low T"). The advertising suggests that reduced libido, lower energy levels, and other symptoms may be indicators of low T. Mind you, there is no medical condition known as "low T." It is the creation of Madison Avenue advertising agencies that realize the market potential in promising the restoration of youthful vitality to aging baby boomers. Yet major pharmaceutical companies have come to the rescue with testosterone gels.

These drugs are already generating more than $2 billion in sales annually.[62] As the population ages over the coming decade, the market for such products could increase dramatically. What's most concerning is that not only are they of highly questionable value, but their long-term adverse effects are not well understood. There is concern that they may enlarge the prostate, as well as increase the likelihood of cardiovascular disease.[63]

Another prime example of this phenomenon can be seen in the advertising for the use of antidepressants to treat social-anxiety disorder. Based on the frequency of the ads, one might conclude that every third person is so afflicted. Nothing could be further from the truth.

There is no empirical, clinical signpost defining social-anxiety disorder. Like most psychiatric conditions, it is diagnosed based on a preponderance of symptoms defined within the DSM-5 (the fifth edition of the *Diagnostic and Statistical Manual of Mental Disorders*, which serves as the Bible for mental-health professionals when they assign a diagnosis to a patient). There is considerable debate as to the incidence rate of social-anxiety disorder, with estimates ranging as low as 1 percent of the population.

Attention-deficit disorder (ADD) is another condition that psychiatry pounced on and arguably overmedicated. In the 1990s, it seemed like every male child in America was a candidate for an ADD or ADHD (attention-deficit hyperactivity disorder) diagnosis. Of course, pharma was close at hand with medications to bring relief—potent stimulants that carried risks of dependency and other problems. ADD and ADHD were economic boons to psychiatrists and the drug industry.

It's not just our minds that get unnecessary medications. It could be our limbs—as in the case of restless-leg syndrome (RLS). There is no definitive diagnosis for this condition. Exactly when does too much leg motion become *restless*? That probably depends on whether you stand to economically benefit, as do pharmaceutical manufacturers of drugs that address RLS.

But these efforts to gin up sales, though far from harmless, are far more benign than capitalizing on people facing life-threatening or debilitating illness, such as cancer patients.

TAKING ADVANTAGE OF PEOPLE AT THEIR MOST VULNERABLE: CANCER PATIENTS

There are few diagnoses that impart a greater sense of vulnerability than cancer. All of us have witnessed it strike close to home—sometimes with dizzying speed and devastating finality. At other times, we watch as our friends or loved ones endure a tense but momentary brush with death but then return to some semblance of health.

Cancer patients, particularly early in their diagnosis, are seeking one thing—a reprieve from the sentence they've been given. That reprieve, if it arrives in time, comes thanks to one or more of three methods of treatment: surgery (cut it out), radiation (burn it out), or chemotherapy (poison it). In addition to each of these treatment modalities, patients may be given an armamentarium of drugs to manage the side effects of cancer treatment.

These drugs represent tremendous sources of revenue for pharmaceutical and biotechnology companies. One example can be seen in promotion of a drug known as Procrit, which purportedly addressed the anemia that results from some forms of chemotherapy by increasing the production of hemoglobin.

Johnson & Johnson, the drug's manufacturer, promoted it using ads that "depicted heartwarming scenes in which cancer patients spoke of the drug's miraculous ability to restore the 'strength for living' that had been drained by cancer chemotherapy."[64] The problem, according to cancer expert Brawley, was that "pharmaceutical companies were promoting an untested therapy that was purported to make patients feel better and stronger when, in fact, it caused strokes and heart attacks and in some cases made tumors grow. My colleagues didn't object. The vast majority of physicians treating cancer were prescribing these drugs and benefiting handsomely from doing so."[65]

Inspired by the success of Procrit, other manufacturers soon introduced competing products. Through aggressive marketing to medical oncologists, including cash incentives for prescribing the drug, Amgen was able to gain market share and grow profits for one of their drugs. Brawley says that he "obtained a copy of a 2006 supply agreement between Amgen and an oncology practice. This is a proprietary document that doesn't circulate widely, and you can see why. It states that a practice that made a gross purchase of $422,800 worth of Aranesp in a single quarter stood to get back 18 percent of that amount—$76,100—in a rebate."[66]

So despite the profound lack of evidence supporting the drug makers' claims, this category of drugs became "the largest-selling class of drugs used in oncology, with 2006 gross sales of 4.85 billion in the United States alone. That year, worldwide sales were $10 billion."[67]

These prescribing patterns morally outraged some physicians, including Brawley, who says that "these drugs were not used to cure disease or make patients feel better. They were used to make money for doctors and pharmaceutical companies at the expense of patients, insurance companies, and taxpayers."[68]

Procrit and Aranesp pale in cost when compared to the latest complex chemotherapy and biologic agents, some of which can be quite efficacious in treating cancer. A drug for treating leukemia, "Gleevec entered the market in 2001 at a price of about $30,000 a year in the United States. . . . Since then, the price has tripled . . . even as Gleevec has faced competition from five newer drugs. And those drugs are even more expensive."[69] It does not take a tremendous volume of patients to hit a home run in sales. In 2012, Gleevec became the top-selling drug at Novartis—racking up $4.7 billion in sales.[70]

Granted, pharmaceutical companies incur tremendous expense when bringing these new compounds to market. There may be an initial investment of $50- to $100 million in research, followed by even larger amounts spent on marketing once the agent is approved. These companies would not make such investments based on altruism. Rather, each new drug represents a tremendous profit opportunity—for example, more than 90 percent of the newly FDA-approved cancer treatments rolled out in 2012 cost more than $100,000 per year, per patient.[71]

The prices of these drugs raise profound ethical questions regarding the value placed on extra weeks, months, or years of life gained through these therapies. This is an issue that both individuals and society as a whole must struggle with.

For the patient fortunate enough to enjoy a relatively symptom-free, prolonged remission, the value may be immense. However, for the advanced colon cancer patient who has no real chance of recovering and is consumed by pain, the $17,000 spent monthly on a chemotherapeutic agent that may do little to forestall death seems more questionable.

Another challenge facing cancer patients is the differential in out-of-pocket costs for oral medications versus chemotherapeutic or biologic agents that are infused. The patient often pays a vastly greater portion of the cost when the drugs are administered orally, offsetting the benefit of some seemingly lower-priced agents.

Temozolomide is one such example. This agent, when used in combination with other therapies, may help prolong the life of patients afflicted with glioblastomas—a particularly insidious and incurable form of brain cancer. Though the six additional months of life "enjoyed," on average, by such patients may seem somewhat paltry, it represents an approximately 50 percent gain in average survival time from diagnosis. Temozolomide, while not inexpensive (approximately $3,000 to $4,000 a month), is far less than drugs such as Erbitux. But because Temozolomide is administered orally, it may cost patients hundreds of dollars per month in copays—money they simply don't have.

Fortunately, numerous states are either considering or have adopted some form of legislation similar to the Cancer Treatment Fairness Act of Florida that would eliminate this discrepancy in out-of-pocket costs for orally administered versus infused drugs for cancer patients.

The best way to battle the arguable profiteering on cancer patients is for physicians to stand up and lead the charge for more-equitable pricing. That's exactly what has begun to happen. A group of leading oncologists recently pressured pharma to reduce its costs: "With the cost of some lifesaving cancer drugs exceeding $100,000 a year, more than one hundred influential cancer specialists from around the world have taken the unusual step of banding together in hopes of persuading some leading pharmaceutical companies to bring prices down."[72]

BUYING CONGRESS

Pharma seeks to buy influence wherever it can—and few places are easier than Washington, D.C. The defense industry was legendary for using lobbyists to increase congressional defense budgets while helping to consummate expensive contracts with the industry. Yet those efforts pale by comparison to what has occurred within health care.

In 2001, consumer watchdog group Public Citizen published some eye-opening statistics about lobbying by the drug industry:

- "The drug industry spent $262 million on political influence in the 1999–2000 election cycle: $177 million on lobbying, $65 million on issue ads, and $20 million on campaign contributions."[73]
- The industry hired 625 different lobbyists last year to buttonhole lawmakers—or more than one lobbyist for every member of Congress. The bill for this team of lobbyists in 2000 alone: $92.3 million."[74]

Things have not changed much over the ensuing decade, according to a report published by OpenSecrets.org, which estimates that "total annual lobbying in 2012 for pharmaceuticals and health products, which includes medical products, dietary and nutritional supplements, etc., equals $234,104,389."[75] Major trade-association Pharmaceutical Research and Manufacturers of America spent $18,530,000. Eli Lilly was second at $11,096,000.[76]

Though not technically defined as *lobbying*, political contributions for 2012 increased to nearly $50 million—up from under $5 million in 1990.[77] In 2012, the average contribution to a Republican member of Congress was in excess of $32,000 and to a Democratic member in excess of $25,000.[78]

Arguably, these efforts have contributed to the preservation of aberrantly high pricing for the drugs that Americans buy and or far less scrutiny of an industry that may be guilty of egregious acts.

PHARMA PROVES IMPERVIOUS TO PAIN

I once had a cat that seemed impervious to pain. When it behaved in an outrageous fashion, it received a swift but tempered punishment designed to dissuade such behaviors. The quick swats had zero impact on my cat (maybe I should have put him in time-out). Pharma appears to respond similarly:

- "Less than three years ago, Novartis settled criminal and civil investigations into whether it promoted drugs to health care professionals for uses not approved by the Food and Drug Administration. It paid $422.5 million to settle the case."[79]
- "Last week, Preet Bharara, the United States attorney for the Southern District of New York, announced the filing of a lawsuit accusing the company of providing even more blatant kickbacks to pharmacies to generate sales of one of its better-selling drugs. The federal prosecutors also filed a second suit, charging that Novartis Pharmaceuticals made illegal payments to physicians in the form of honorariums and other benefits to induce them to write prescriptions for various drugs made by the company."[80]
- "Last year GlaxoSmithKline paid the largest health fraud settlement ever, a hefty $3 billion, and two other companies paid $1.5 billion or more."[81]

Perhaps to pharma such fines are simply the cost of doing business and are already fully factored into their pricing.

As with other topics in this book, there is much more ground to be covered relative to the abuses perpetrated by the pharmaceutical industry. Furthermore, it should be acknowledged that many, similar, issues arise when investigating the medical-device industry.

WHAT YOU CAN DO TO PROTECT YOUR HEALTH

Though it may be difficult, if not impossible, to protect yourself from falsified research regarding drugs that you may be prescribed, there is nonetheless a great deal you can do to safeguard your health and the health of your family.

Trust in God, but from Your Physician Demand Proof

The first step is to make certain that you are comfortable with your physicians—particularly your primary care physician—and how, when, and why he or she recommends certain drugs. There are three critical elements that underlie such trust: (1) the knowledge or belief that your physician's judgment is unaffected by industry relationships, (2) the evidence that your physician stays current on the medical research and literature and read studies with a discerning eye, and (3) the certainty that your physician welcomes your scrutiny and active stewardship of your health.

A good place to begin is by researching your physician's prescribing patterns. Until recently, no one, not even your physician, had ready access to such powerful data. But thanks to the not-for-profit consumer advocacy group ProPublica, much of that information now resides in a Web-accessible repository.

ProPublica relied on the Freedom of Information Act to obtain pre-scribing data from the Centers for Medicare and Medicaid Services (CMS). Though it took time and wrangling, CMS turned over not only data on all prescriptions written under Medicare Part D by the nation's physicians but also information on state-by-state prescribing patterns and associated costs.[82]

Once properly structured to facilitate easy access and interpretation, the data allowed researchers and consumers to see at a glance how a given physician compared to his or her peers in prescribing patterns. One could quickly discern a doctor's most frequently prescribed drugs, the number of prescriptions by drug with associated costs, and how these patterns compared to other physicians in the state or in his or her specialty.

"What we found was disturbing," said the study's authors. "Although we did not have access to patient names or medical records, it was clear that hundreds of physicians across the country were prescribing large numbers of dangerous, inappropriate, or unnecessary drugs."[83] They provided numerous examples, including the observation that "among the top prescribers of the most-abused painkillers, we found many who had been charged with crimes, convicted, disciplined by their state medical boards, or terminated from state Medicaid programs for the poor. But nearly all remained eligible to prescribe to Medicare patients."[84]

So whether you are checking into the prescribing patterns of your existing physician or researching the habits of a doctor to whom you've been referred, the data may prove illuminating. Remember, you may now know more than your physician does about what he or she jots down on that small white pad many times each day.

If you have doubts about whether your physician is receiving funding from related industries, look them up on the Internet. A number of prestigious institutions began publishing this data early, including Duke's Clinical Research Institute. Pharmaceutical companies like Eli Lilly were also quick to promise publication on their websites. Remember, the Physician Payments Sunshine Act has resulted in the broad dissemination of this information in 2014: "The Patient Protection and Affordable Health Care Act (H.R. 3590) signed into law in March 2010 includes the Physician Payments Sunshine Act (section 6002) (PPSA), which requires pharmaceutical, medical-device, biological, and medical-supply manufacturers to report to Health and Human Services (HHS) any 'payment or other transfer of value' to physicians and teaching hospitals. The first reports will be due March 31, 2013, for the calendar year 2012 reporting period."[85]

The Dangers Lurking in Your Medicine Cabinet

Next, you need to take inventory of all the prescription drugs you and your family are taking (or have been prescribed). This list should also include a list of over-the-counter (OTC) medications, herbal supplements, nutriceuticals, or other "alternative" medicines. The list should be methodically reviewed with your physician during your annual physical, if not before. During that review, provide your doctor with their own copy of the list. Here are some of the questions you then need to pose:

- Why am I on each of these medications, and are there medications that I could discontinue or be safely weaned from at this time?

- Are there any negative, synergistic interactions between these drugs—or between the prescription medications and my OTC, herbal, or other alternative medicines?
- Are any of these drugs particularly dangerous or potentially injurious to my health? Discuss each one with a doctor and get second opinions. Information is also available online at trusted sources.

It may be helpful for you to do a bit of your own research before having this conversation. It is relatively simple to look up any drug. The Web is your best bet for fast information. However, be a bit wary of the websites established by the pharmaceutical manufacturers of the drug—though their content is regulated, the site is still designed to sell you on the benefits of the drug. Here are a few sites that are definitely worth investigating:

- MedlinePlus's Drugs, Supplements, and Herbal Information page (a service of the U.S. National Library of Medicine and National Institutes of Health)[86]
- Drugs.com (commercial site with consumer-friendly information)[87]
- WebMD (commercial site with consumer-friendly information)[88]
- the FDA's Drugs website (very technical but timely information)[89]
- Mayo Clinic's Drugs and Supplements site (excellent site from one of America's most trusted providers)[90]
- CVS's Drug Information Center (CVS and Walgreen both sponsor sites containing valuable information)[91]
- Natural Medicine's Comprehensive Database, Consumer Version (a great source of objective information on herbals and other remedies)[92]
- The FDA's Health-Fraud Scams page (provides valuable information on how to be a more discerning health care consumer)[93]

These sites will help you discern a number of critical facts about your medications, including

- the indications for using a particular drug;
- warnings associated with the drug—from contraindications for taking it to potentially fatal side effects;

- synergistic interactions with other drugs, herbals, and food products;
- general information that may be helpful to anyone on the medication—particularly if it is for a chronic (versus acute) condition; and
- other drugs in the same class that may have a different side-effect profile or be available as a generic.

Don't try to become a physician or pharmacist. Simply become an informed consumer. You may find that something as seemingly innocuous as garlic can seriously interfere with your diabetes medication.

Once you and your physicians complete the review, it will be important to keep your list up to date. Whenever a new drug is prescribed or you start taking an OTC medication or alternative medicine, be sure to log it.

OTC and Other Terrorizing Compounds

Many consumers assume that over-the-counter drugs are completely safe or they would not be available without prescription. Nothing could be further from the truth. Many OTC products are quite potent and must be taken in the dosages recommended to avoid toxicity. Acetaminophen, the active ingredient in Tylenol, is a perfect example. When properly administered, it is a wonderful mild analgesic. However, in excessively high dosages or when combined indiscriminately with alcohol, it can cause serious liver damage.

Above a certain threshold, virtually every OTC drug is poisonous. Therefore good judgment must be used when taking them. The same principle applies to a myriad of herbal remedies, vitamins, and alternative medicines that the majority of Americans consume. Though we may spend more than $26 billion each year on these products, most consumers are unaware of the risks associated with certain compounds.

Some compounds are dangerous due to poor manufacturing processes that may leave them contaminated with toxic chemicals. Contamination may be particularly problematic with compounds imported from countries like China that have lax consumer-safety protocols. Others are inherently dangerous due to their impact on our physiology. Remember, the FDA does not force its stringent protective rules on nonprescription products . . . so to some degree you are at the mercy of the manufacturer.

Consumer Reports lists what it refers to as the *dirty dozen*—twelve of the most dangerous supplements: aconite, bitter orange, chaparral, colloidal silver, coltsfoot, comfrey, country mallow, germanium, greater celandine, kava, lobelia, and yohimbe.[94] You'll find many of these ingredients still on the market, despite their lurking dangers.

Not Falling Prey to Propaganda

You cannot watch television for long without encountering suggestions about how to fix your erectile dysfunction, clear your skin of psoriasis, or get your heart back to a natural rhythm. Direct-to-consumer advertising for pharmaceuticals may have diminished from its all-time high, but it still permeates the airwaves.

I can see virtually no value to the patient in listening to these advertisements. If you trust your physician, then trust that he or she knows what medicines you need to treat specific conditions. Don't be pulled in by warm images of couples canoeing across a pastoral lake at sunset or grandfathers enjoying a day of fishing with their grandsons. Marketers know that when they cannot appeal to logic, they can still appeal to your heart. Forge an emotional connection, and you might be well on your way to selling your drug.

There's No Free Lunch

Finally, and perhaps most importantly, realize that virtually every drug you take comes with a price that transcends what you pay out of pocket. Side effects can range from simply annoying to simply dead . . . even with "all-natural" products. Hemlock is "all natural," but it killed Socrates.

MYTH 8
"I'M JUST THE PATIENT; I'M NOT PART OF THE PROBLEM"

Sarah Matthews had always struggled with her weight. Her life was a series of disappointing attempts to control her insatiable appetite. It came at a hefty price—to her self-esteem, her relationships, and ultimately to her health.

Though her physician had long counseled her to lose weight and begin to exercise, Sarah continued her habit of consuming more than four thousand calories a day. Her weight at age forty-two had swelled to more than 280 pounds, and her joints were showing the wear of carrying such a big burden.

But it was more than Sarah's joints that were beginning to fail. Her annual physical revealed that she was perilously close to becoming a full-blown diabetic. Her blood pressure hovered at 160/100, which is very high, and the slightest exertion made her short of breath. At this pace, Sarah's life would be dramatically shortened. As a diabetic, she would run the risk of blindness, loss of limbs, and eventually death. If her blood pressure remained high, coronary-artery disease would naturally follow—potentially precipitating a stroke or heart attack. Furthermore, recently published research suggested that the earlier one becomes obese, the greater the probability of developing atherosclerosis.

This time, her physician was unflinching in his strongly worded advice: "Lose the weight now. There are no more tomorrows." Sarah broke down in tears. It was not a lack of desire to lose weight; she simply didn't know how to win the battle against her lifelong demon. Fortunately, her physician had a dedicated nurse educator, who not only started Sarah on the path to recovery but enlisted the help of a counselor, a nutritionist, and an exercise coach.

Frightened by the prospect of a grim future, Sarah became compliant. Though it took more than a year, she successfully shed just shy of one hundred pounds through daily diet and exercise. Her lab values responded in tandem with her changes in lifestyle. After eighteen long, difficult months, Sarah was able to stop taking her medications. What appeared to be the beginning of a lifelong path of advancing chronic illness had been stopped in its tracks.

TAKING PERSONAL RESPONSIBILITY FOR OUR BEHAVIOR

The message emblazoned in every chapter of this book has been that our health care system has gross deficiencies that can seriously affect your care. Numerous strategies have been outlined about how to increase the probability of receiving the "right" care for you and your family. *Yet the best strategy of all is to simply not need care in the first place.*

That means taking exquisitely good care of ourselves—a lesson that Sarah is learning late in life. Sarah was not merely the patient. She was also the problem. It was her eating behavior—not some random disease or virus—that was causing her to develop debilitating, chronic conditions. Had she maintained her current trajectory, these conditions could have robbed her of joy, health, and ultimately her life. In the process, Sarah would have required an increasing onslaught of medications and other interventions, all of which would have brought their own associated risks and contributed to feeding the national health care bill.

Granted, not all of us seem to suffer the ill effects of an unhealthy lifestyle. Some people get away with murder when it comes to their bodies. My mother was one such person. Finding the best restaurants and bakeries was a lifelong passion for her, though she somehow stayed slim. Her idea of strenuous exercise was a full day of shopping. Her habits finally caught up with her at the age of sixty-five, though, when her severely blocked arteries necessitated quadruple-bypass surgery. Having her chest brutally cracked open slowed her down for a short time, but before long she was back to her diet of candy, cookies, fried chicken, and steaks.

My mother's diet contributed to her development of cardiovascular disease (including a heart attack), transient-ischemic events (TIAs—or "mini-strokes"), and insulin-dependent diabetes. Despite her multiple comorbidities, she lived another twenty-two years and seemed to enjoy almost every minute.

There are always exceptions, but poor lifestyle choices eventually catch up with most of us, taking a major toll on our health and well-being. Whether it is smoking, overindulging in food or alcohol, or fool-ishly taking chances with drugs, promiscuous sexual behavior, or the need for speed when behind the wheel of an automobile, our choices often determine our fates.

Proof can be found in the data collected by the Centers for Disease Control (CDC), who keep close tabs on our nation's health. The CDC's website contains some startling illustrations of the impact of lifestyle choices on the health of the population:

- Seven out of ten deaths among Americans each year are from chronic diseases. Heart disease, cancer, and stroke account for more than 50 percent of all deaths each year.
- In 2005, 133 million Americans—almost one out of every two adults—had at least one chronic illness.
- Obesity has become a major health concern. One in every three adults is obese, and almost one in five youths between the ages of six and nineteen is obese.
- Diabetes continues to be the leading cause of kidney failure, non-traumatic lower-extremity amputations, and blindness among adults age twenty to seventy-four.
- Excessive alcohol consumption is the third leading preventable cause of death in the United States behind diet, physical activity, and tobacco.[1]

The bottom line is that we are a chronically ill nation and our ill-nesses are not merely debilitating but also costly—resulting in hundreds of billions of dollars spent unnecessarily on health care expenditures every year. And the situation is deteriorating!

It doesn't have to be this way. We have the power to change our nation's prognosis. Many of the chronic diseases we experience are either preventable or can be delayed until the latter stages of our life. This simple yet profound message was preached for more than thirty years by Dr. James Fries. The question is, Do we have the will to change?

COMPRESSION OF MORBIDITY: A FANCY TERM FOR A SIMPLE GOAL

The July 17, 1980, issue of the *New England Journal of Medicine* featured a landmark article by Jim Fries, MD, professor of medicine at Stanford University. The article became one of the most frequently cited scientific references in the emerging field of wellness. Fries focused on the impact of chronic disease, which he described as "responsible for more than 80 percent of all deaths and for an even higher fraction of cases of total disability. Arteriosclerosis (including coronary-artery disease and stroke), arthritis, adult-onset diabetes, chronic obstructive-pulmonary disease (including emphysema), cancer, and cirrhosis represent the overwhelming majority of our health problems. They are widespread conditions that originate in early life and develop insidiously; the probability of their occurrence increases with age."[2]

Fries's contribution did not lie in describing the inescapable spiral of chronic disease into disability and death. Rather, it was his challenging theory of the "compression of morbidity" that suggested the progression of disease and infirmity could be forestalled. "Disability and lowered quality of life due to the most prevalent chronic diseases are thus inescapably linked with eventual mortality," he wrote. "These chronic diseases are approached most effectively with a strategy of 'postponement' rather than cure. If the rate of progression is decreased, then the date of passage through the clinical threshold is postponed; if sufficiently postponed, the symptomatic threshold may not be crossed during a lifetime, and the disease is 'prevented.'"[3]

Fries is stating that, while we cannot escape the human condition, by taking care of ourselves we can stay vital, active, and healthy until the very twilight of our lives. In Fries's mind, that would be living the good life. He even went so far as to point to behavior changes that would compress morbidity, saying that "some chronic illnesses definitely can be postponed; elimination of cigarette smoking greatly delays the date of onset of symptoms of emphysema and reduces the probability of lung cancer. Treatment of hypertension retards development of certain complications in the arteries. In other illnesses, circumstantial evidence of similar effects of postponement is strong, but proof is difficult: that arteriosclerosis is retarded by weight reduction or exercise is suggested by associative data but has not yet been proven."[4]

I was fortunate enough to meet Jim Fries when he was part of a panel assembled by my mentor, Martin Seligman, at the University of Pennsylvania. Seligman, who was working under a Robert Wood Johnson Foundation grant, had assembled some of the brightest minds in preventative medicine to define the emerging field of positive health, including Dr. Fries. Fries obviously lives by the tenets he preaches, for he appeared to be in great physical condition.

In the intervening three-plus decades since Fries published this article, our knowledge on wellness and prevention has expanded greatly. Thousands of researchers have built on Fries's foundational research, and the accumulated knowledge provides us with powerful but disheartening information on the degree to which our population is managing their lifestyle behaviors to affect wellness:

- More than one-third of all adults do not meet recommendations for aerobic physical activity based on the 2008 Physical Activity Guidelines for Americans, and 23 percent report no leisure-time physical activity at all in the preceding month.
- More than forty-three million American adults smoke. Lung cancer is the leading cause of cancer death, and cigarette smoking causes almost all cases.
- Excessive alcohol consumption contributes to over fifty-four different diseases and injuries.[5]

If you are wondering how that compares to other people in other nations, "in terms of individual behaviors, Americans are less likely to smoke and may drink less heavily than their counterparts in peer countries, but they consume the most calories per capita, abuse more prescription and illicit drugs, are less likely to fasten seatbelts, have more traffic accidents involving alcohol, and own more firearms than their peers in other countries."[6] As we saw in the opening chapter of this book, our nation pays dearly for its behavior as evidenced by our poor population health status relative to every other industrialized nation.

Regardless of one's nationality, the trick is not in knowing merely what to modify but how to modify our behaviors so that we live longer, happier, healthier lives.

A PSYCHIATRIST'S ADVICE: GET OFF THE COUCH!

John Ratey, professor of Psychiatry at Harvard Medical School, wrote one of the most motivating books I have read on wellness. *Spark* is a highly readable text describing the profound changes that occur within our brains and bodies with regular aerobic exercise.

Though not a panacea for all that ails us, exercise comes closer to a health-inducing tonic than any other intervention, according to Ratey, and he provides the data to support his argument. Regular, sustained aerobic exercise improves our mind's ability to learn, decreases negative emotions, impulsivity, and addictions, and bolsters overall health by countering the effects of stress and aging.[7]

I was introduced to Dr. Ratey's work by Ray Fowler, PhD, the former president of the American Psychological Association. Ray's personal story is an interesting one. According to Fowler, he was a self-described couch potato much of his adult life. Fearing the long-term consequences of a laissez-faire attitude toward health, Ray got off the couch in his fifties and started to run.

Mere running was not enough for Ray. He set the seemingly unattainable goal of running in the Boston Marathon within one year. Dr. Fowler was overweight, accustomed to a sedentary lifestyle, and had just begun to jog. Yet those who know Fowler were little surprised when he actually pulled it off.

When I met Ray, he was in his late seventies and still amazingly fit. Each day he walked a bare minimum of ten thousand paces. It was his ritual, and he loved to bring others into his walking club. Each night at midnight, a group of world-class psychologists and researchers would check in to ensure that each had completed their exercise. Most members of the "club" were in their sixties or seventies, and all were eager to outdo one another.

The APA has honored Ray's many contributions by holding a race during their annual conference. Today their website notes that "Ray's Race was named in honor of Dr. Ray Fowler, former APA CEO and founder of the Running Psychologists in 1979. We encourage runners and walkers of all ages and levels of ability to participate in the race."[8]

Fowler and Ratey have much in common. They know the power of the mind-body connection and that wellness and well-being go hand in hand. They also know that the most powerful "medication" one can prescribe is exercise. By example, Ratey describes studies demonstrating that regular aerobic exercise is equally efficacious in treating mild to moderate depression as are powerful medications . . . without the costs, side effects, or potential perceived loss of self-efficacy associated with surrendering control to a pill.

Why don't physicians follow Fowler's and Ratey's advice and put their patients on a prescription of aerobic exercise versus SSRIs for their mild to moderate depression? I posed this question to a physician at Saint Luke's who had long championed wellness initiatives. Though he concurred with the statement that frequent aerobic exercise of sufficient duration was equally efficacious as SSRIs in treating mild to moderate depression, he said it would be exceedingly difficult to change physician prescribing patterns. When I pushed him on why physicians would prefer an intervention that consumed resources, carried the risks of side effects, and limited a patient's perceived self-efficacy, he said, "It's easier." Several mental-health providers with whom I subsequently spoke agreed with this assertion.

They are right. It's far easier for physicians to write scripts and certainly far easier for patients to pop the pills. But is it the right thing to do?

For many patients, the very nature of their depression may make participating in a new exercise ritual an overwhelming challenge, while other patients may find that exercise proves to be a potent and welcome ally in reducing their depressive symptoms. The right path for each patient should be determined through a collaborative and informed conversation with their physician.

Exercise affects far more than mood and cognition. A recently released research study conducted by the Epidemiology Research Program at the American Cancer Society reveals a strong correlation between regular aerobic exercise (in particular, walking) and a marked reduction in the risk of developing breast cancer in postmenopausal women. Those women who exercised most vigorously appeared to realize as much as a 25 percent decrease in their risk of developing cancer.[9]

WHERE TO GO FROM HERE: BEGIN WITH A HEALTH RISK ASSESSMENT

If you are ready to step forward and assume stewardship responsibility for your health and well-being, then congratulations! You've made a life-altering decision. But before you hit the jogging trails or straddle an elliptical trainer, there are a few things you may wish to consider—beginning with establishing your current health status (and risks). Not only will this help you formulate a personal health plan, but it will also provide you with a gauge by which to measure your progress.

One of the simplest ways to determine your health status is by completing a health risk assessment (HRA). An HRA is a questionnaire used to provide a glimpse into your overall health and well-being. A relatively comprehensive HRA will address such issues as

- biometric indicators of your current health status, including blood-glucose levels, blood pressure, serum cholesterol, weight, and waist circumference—all potential risk factors relative to developing chronic conditions;
- diagnosed medical conditions;
- family history of major diseases where there may be a genetic propensity to develop that disease;
- lifestyle behaviors that increase your risk of injury or illness;
- lifestyle behaviors that decrease such risk;
- perceived stress levels; and
- perceived well-being and life satisfaction.

HRAs often group respondents into one of four categories that move progressively from left to right according to increased morbidity. Therefore, at the far left are the optimally well, and at the far right are the chronically ill. As Fries taught us, everyone progresses from left to right . . . the question is *at what pace?* The HRA often points out specific areas that a consumer can focus on to improve their score. It may also link to a repository of tools and other resources designed to help the respondent slow his or her movement from one risk category to another.

HRAs have become ubiquitous among many corporations providing health care benefits to their employees. Employers want their employed population to remain healthy—because beyond any altruistic benefits, lowered frequency of illness and injury reduces the cost burden of insuring them, while also improving productivity. More and more employers are incentivizing their workforce to complete HRAs (often with an accompanying annual physical that provides the biometric data). At Saint Luke's Health System, half the cost of our employer-sponsored health insurance was covered if we were compliant with these simple mandates.

HRAs are not without controversy. Employees at various organizations, including Penn State, have raised serious objections to being "coerced" into completing the assessments through the use of monetary penalties for failure to comply. Employees and their representatives have voiced concern over how confidential health status information might be used punitively by the employer. These concerns are valid. Even so, I am willing to trade off what I believe to be a minor risk for a major gain in understanding about my health status.

University of Michigan researcher Dee Edington demonstrated that the mere act of completing an HRA reduced an employee's risk score. Presumably this was attributable to heightened awareness on the part of the employee about their level of risk and the degree to which it could be self-regulated. Even if an employee's health simply remains stable, there is a strong economic value, according to Edington. In fact, "Edington Associates cites data showing that simply maintaining an employee's health can save up to $1,500 a year compared with the average costs associated with an employee whose health continues to decline."[10]

If you are retired, don't worry; you don't have to be in the workforce to benefit from an HRA. Medicare beneficiaries can also take advantage of a free HRA, thanks to the Affordable Care Act, which "requires that a health risk assessment be included in the annual wellness visit benefit authorized for Medicare beneficiaries under the act."[11]

It should be noted that HRAs are not a substitute for your annual wellness exam conducted by a primary care physician or nurse practitioner. Your physician should be an excellent source of information about how to improve your health status as well as what type of exercise regimens might be most appropriate for you.

Some primary care practices are embracing a new model of care that emphasizes wellness and prevention. Known as the *medical home*, such practices are designed to reduce unnecessary utilization through better health management. Nurse educators play an important role in working with patients to improve their wellness and well-being. If you do not currently have a primary care physician, you may wish to consider getting one associated with a medical home.

WHY AREN'T HOSPITALS MORE SUPPORTIVE OF WELLNESS?

In a word, *money*. The current economic incentives are for the provision of expensive services—not for maximizing the health of patients.

While working for a major health system, I sought to enlist the support of my colleagues on the senior-leadership team for an aggressive wellness initiative targeted at major employers in our market. Most of my colleagues could not get past the seemingly oxymoronic nature of doing everything in our power to reduce an employed population's need for our services. I explained that not only was this our moral obligation, but it would also prove to be a great business strategy in the long run.

I had tested this theory with senior executives in major corporations. My pitch to them was simple: *Our health system's job is to do everything in our power to keep your employees healthy and out of our health system. When they must receive care, our job is to deliver the most effective and efficient care possible.* One of our region's largest employers said in response, "If you can deliver on that promise, you'll have 100 percent of our business."

I still believe had we pursued this strategy and honored both elements of our value proposition that our health system would have stood to gain tremendous market advantage . . . and would have done so in a commendable manner that was based not on marketing hyperbole but on good work.

However, I strongly believe that for the hospital industry to broadly embrace wellness it will require a transition from its current fee-for-service reimbursement method to a payment mechanism aligned with the goal of longitudinal-care management that optimizes the health and well-being of patients.

SAYING THE SERENITY PRAYER

The HRA identifies both risk factors that are within our ability to control and ones that are independent of it. It is essential to remember that some aspects of our health and well-being are completely beyond our control. They may be influenced by unavoidable exposure to viruses, diseases, or environmental toxins. They may result from an unforeseen accident. Or they may also be hardwired into our genes and waiting for the right moment or trigger to unfold. For those factors that we cannot control, we can nonetheless behave like knowledgeable and appropriate consumers of health care resources—doing our part to reduce the unnecessary or inappropriate overuse of medical interventions.

GENETIC TESTING: THE NEW FRONTIER

Our understanding of the role that genetics play in disease development and progression is advancing at a blindingly fast pace. We are on the cusp of a scientific revolution that will change the face of medicine as we know it. In the near future, physicians will be able to identify how our individual genetic makeups predispose each of us to a wide range of conditions. This knowledge will empower us to better maintain our health by focusing on preventing or delaying diseases to which we are most susceptible. It will also enable the development of personalized treatments that address the impact of our aberrant genes. In the coming decades, cytotoxic chemotherapies may largely give way to vastly more effective and less toxic targeted therapies. Hopefully these therapies will be priced in a manner that renders them accessible to those in need.

We've already seen how BRAC1-positive women, whose likelihood of developing breast cancer may be as high as 80 percent, may be spared a dire fate by electing to have prophylactic mastectomies. Similarly, the knowledge that we are destined to develop diabetes, coronary-artery disease, or other conditions might cause us to aggressively embrace certain prevention practices.

A growing number of companies can provide you with significant insight into an expanding number of genetic conditions for which you may carry a key mutation. The tests are simple, anonymous, and done via the mail. The knowledge you glean, however, may be anything but simple—particularly if it brings difficult news. For instance, you may learn of a genetic predisposition for a potentially devastating condition for which there are no current cures, such as Alzheimer's. Or you may learn that you have passed along a defective gene to one of your children, thus imperiling their health. That's why a number of the more reputable testing firms offer a counseling service to complement their testing. That's also why, in November 2013, the FDA began investigating the marketing practices of some genetic-testing firms.

WHEN YOUR HEALTH OR WELL-BEING IS COMPROMISED

Prevention is critically important. There are times, however, when you must interface with the health care system. Your job, at those moments, is to be a prudent steward of health care resources. That means seeking out the most efficient and effective methods of restoring your health. It implies a high level of awareness of the expensive diagnostic or treatment modalities that the system will be more than happy to provide you.

In the case of a relatively minor injury, your first impulse may be to rush for an MRI when a simple examination or X-ray will more than suffice. If the pain persists, you may be motivated to seek out a quick surgical "solution," when watchful waiting will achieve an equal if not better outcome in the long run.

If you are wondering how well I practice what I preach, allow me to share two quick stories with you illustrating poor versus proper stewardship.

POOR STEWARDSHIP

Through the years, I've had periodic inner-ear infections that caused dizziness or disequilibrium lasting a few days to a few weeks. The dizziness and vertigo that I experienced a couple years ago was different—it was unremitting.

As time wore on, I became increasing convinced that the dizziness I was experiencing had to be a malignant brain tumor, a malformation of a major blood vessel in my brain, or something equally catastrophic.

When my primary care physicians didn't seem adequately concerned about my condition, I sought out an ear, nose, and throat doctor. When the ENT's examination revealed nothing substantive, the specialist ordered a CT of my inner ear. The results came back negative, and I was back at square one. So I contacted a neurologist friend of mine. Greatly concerned with my well-being, she ordered an MRI of my brain. It, too, came back negative.

Undaunted, I went to a neuroaudiologist seeking an opinion. He examined me thoroughly and ordered multiple tests to reveal potential problems with my inner ear. Once again, the results came back negative. I consulted my favorite neurosurgeon to rule out any relationship between my symptoms and issues with my neck. He assured me that there was little likelihood that my past neck problems correlated with my present dizziness.

In desperation, I returned to my PCP; he recommended I have my eyes checked.

A new pair of glasses provided a new lease on life and much relief to my dizziness. In the process of discovering the culprit behind my malady, I had expended thousands of dollars in health care resources and delayed a solution to my problem. The good news was that there was no brain tumor. The bad news was that I had abused the privilege of being able to access our health care system by demanding services that I really didn't need.

PROPER STEWARDSHIP

Several summers ago, I was at the lake waterskiing with my son and his buddies. It was early in the season and my first day up on skis. As the throttle of the boat belted out an echoing groan, I felt the four hundred–horsepower engine propelling me out of the water. The only problem was that the tips of my skis were pointed in opposite directions. Those of you who ski know that this is a prescription for disaster—particularly if you insist on not letting go of the towrope under the false belief that you can defy physics.

I was far too proud to let go and watched as my legs did the splits. The popping sound of a large muscle being torn from its bony mooring was so loud that I could hear it above the din of the engine. That's when I dropped the rope. It took a few minutes for the full wave of pain to envelope me. When it did, I knew my skiing days were over for several summers to come.

Over the next week, my skin, beginning at the abdomen and descending below my left knee, turned black from pooled blood. My wife told me that there was probably little anyone could do to repair the injury. Two other physicians, whose specialties made them a bit more in tune to such injuries, rendered the same opinion. Each doctor also offered to order an MRI. When I asked if the results might change the course of treatment, the response was no.

It might have been comforting to have an expensive imaging test that my insurance company paid for, but if it wasn't going to affect the treatment or outcome of my injury, what was the point? Though it took six months, my injury eventually healed without medical intervention. The following summer, I got back up on skis, and I now use a bit more judgment when things seem to be going awry.

WHAT YOU CAN DO TO PROTECT YOUR HEALTH

The starting point on your journey toward wellness is to assess your level of risk. You need to complete or update your HRA, including biometrics. Whoever administers your HRA and biometric screening can provide some preliminary educational material on areas of potential concern.

Your primary care physician should help you define the types of exercise that are appropriate for your current condition. Exercise is not a punishment; therefore your daily trips to the gym should not be drudgery. The key is to find things you enjoy doing. Ideally, you will come up with several exercise routines, each with unique benefits, and alternate your workouts accordingly.

My wife loves Zumba, but she also enjoys the challenge of running. I wouldn't be caught dead in a Zumba class, and running wreaks havoc on my knees. My sport of choice for the past forty years has been tae kwon do. I augment it with aerobic workouts on the elliptical trainer and an aggressive game or two of tennis each week. If you need a jump-start to identify the right workout, sample different classes or consider engaging a personal trainer for a few introductory sessions. When it raises your heartbeat but doesn't feel like work, you've probably found the right exercise. For many if not most people, simply working more walking into your day will do the trick. Park in the last spot from your destination; take the stairs instead of the elevator; walk to do errands when possible.

Next, you need to set your goals as part of a personal-wellness plan. Keep in mind that though the prescription for a healthier and happier life is relatively straightforward, achieving the level of change required to fill that prescription is anything but easy. Your success is contingent on a number of factors:

- Ensure that your goals are realistic and attainable over the period of time you have defined.
- Understand that behavioral change does not occur without resistance and that your journey to wellness may be marked by the proverbial "three steps forward, two steps back." It may help to read what the experts have to say about behavioral change. A good place to begin would be the book *Changing for Good: A Revolutionary Six-Stage Program for Overcoming Bad Habits and Moving Your Life Positively Forward* by James O. Prochaska, John Norcross, and Carlo DiClemente.
- Establish a supportive network that encourages change, whether at work or at home, as did Ray Fowler with his walking group. Remember that nothing will derail your progress faster than a loved one unsupportive of what you are seeking to accomplish. Such lack of support may not manifest as contempt for your process but simply as indulging in behaviors from which you are abstaining.

- Investigate high-tech aids that can keep you on track. When I needed to lose twenty pounds, I installed an app known as My Fitness Pal on my smartphone. It helped me keep track of every calorie I consumed and burned. Because I had to log every bite of food I ingested, it heightened my awareness of overeating.
- Find exercise routines that are fun, not tedious. Varying your routines not only keeps them fresh but also benefits your body by providing different physiological challenges.
- Have an annual physical and participate in age-appropriate screenings (with the caveats enumerated earlier in this book).
- When you momentarily fall off the wagon—and you will—get back on. Setbacks are simply part of the behavioral-change process . . . and human nature. Don't allow momentary indulgences to become defeating daily habits.
- Never be self-deprecating. It is essential that you be kind to yourself as you begin your journey toward wellness.
- Try to avoid being overly rigid while simultaneously being perseverant. When I competed nationally in tae kwon do while in my twenties, I missed out on a lot of fun simply because I was dogmatic about the requirements of my training.
- Celebrate your success! When you achieve those hard-to-reach goals, let others know what you have accomplished. Though you did the work for your own benefit, the external validation nonetheless feels good.

Though a sedentary activity, reading is one of the best ways for you to get energized to live a healthier and more fulfilling life. Just as it is important to fill your stomach with healthy foods, so too must you fill you mind with honest, constructive, and easily understood messages that will contribute to wellness. There are innumerable books on wellness. You might start by considering books by authors Herbert Benson, MD; Dean Ornish, MD; Deepak Chopra; Andrew Weil, MD; Michael Pollan; and, of course, John Ratey.

MYTH 9
"MY INSURANCE COMPANY'S FIRST CONCERN IS MY HEALTH"

In June 2009, the House Energy and Commerce Committee's Oversight and Investigations Subcommittee met to address purported abuses by the insurance industry. The stories the representatives heard during those hearings were mind-boggling. What follows is but one vignette.

A year prior to the hearings, a fifty-nine-year-old retired nurse named Robin Beaton visited her dermatologist for a relatively mundane problem—acne. That would have been the end of it had Ms. Beaton not subsequently developed an aggressive type of breast cancer. [1]

> *Her insurance carrier precertified her for a double mastectomy and hospital stay. But three days before the operation, the insurance company called and told her they had red-flagged her chart and she would not be able to have her surgery.*
>
> *The reason? In May 2008, Beaton had visited a dermatologist for acne. A word written on her chart was interpreted to mean precancerous, so the insurance company decided to launch an investigation into her medical history.* [2]

Despite the protestations of her dermatologist, who stated unequivocally that Ms. Beaton had never had skin cancer, the carrier maintained its denial of coverage. [3] *As Beaton scrambled for a solution to the* *dilemma, not to mention the $30,000 advance payment being demanded by the hospital, time was ticking by, and her tumor was continuing to grow.*

Only after Beaton contacted Texas Representative Joe Barton, who intervened with the president of the insurance carrier, was Beaton's coverage reinstated.[4] *By the time the paperwork had been resolved and surgery performed, Beaton's tumor had more than doubled in size.*[5] *As a result, her surgery was more complicated and her prognosis potentially less promising.*

Robin Beacon held little sway over the insurance company that held her fate in their hands. She may have been the recipient of the intended care, but she was not the one picking up the tab for the service—that was the insurance company's domain. This separation of patient and payer, which clearly influences the care that is delivered to a patient, defines the U.S. health care system. It's a system in which nearly 85 percent of the population, or more than 250 million Americans, have some form of coverage—through either a government-sponsored plan, such as Medicare and Medicaid, or via private insurance.[6]

Robin, like the majority of Americans, was covered by private insurance. Her insurance company operated in a highly competitive market in which both for-profit and not-for-profit companies vied to underwrite covered lives. Like most such companies, it faced the impossible challenge of battling ever-escalating health care bills. It relied on potent weapons in this battle, including denial of charges. In some cases, such denials were absolutely appropriate and protective of the patient and payer. At other times, denials dramatically reduced a patient's odds of surviving or thriving, as was arguably the case with Beacon.

Denial of services is but one tool that private insurance companies rely on to maintain their profitability. Before 2010, companies also relied on lifetime limits on coverage (which could easily be exceeded by a chronic, serious illness) and exorbitant prices for consumers with pre-existing conditions—if such individuals could even obtain coverage in the first place. The most powerful tool, however, was constantly rising premiums.

THE RISING COST OF HEALTH INSURANCE

Escalating premiums are taking a huge bite out of everyone's pocketbook. Health insurance premiums for family coverage dramatically increased from 2000 to 2010—rising 114 percent. What may be even more alarming is the rate of increase in employee contributions during this same period—147 percent![7] According to the Centers for Disease Control (CDC), "in 2000 the average annual premiums for employer-sponsored health insurance were $2,471 for single coverage and $6,438 for family coverage. In 2010, premiums more than doubled to $5,049 for single coverage and $13,770 for family coverage."[8]

A 2007 Institute of Medicine report took note of health care's rising costs on the business community and its implications. The report stated that the financial burden on employers from covering health care costs had increased by 78 percent over the five years prior to the study. Such costs, according to the authors, impaired the global competitiveness of U.S. industry and its products and services.[9]

Though businesses bore the brunt of escalating costs, workers were nonetheless affected due to their premium contributions. According to a 2012 Kaiser Family Foundation survey, "covered workers contribute on average 18 percent of the premium for single coverage and 28 percent of the premium for family coverage."[10]

Not everyone has been penalized equally by rising costs. Just as care varies geographically, so too does the cost of providing health insurance. Research studies have shown an estimated 30 percent variance in cost of insurance among states. The most disturbing finding of this research, however, is that in 2011 health insurance premiums equaled or exceeded 20 percent of a family's annual income in thirty-five states. By comparison, in 2003 only one state met this criterion.[11]

Insurance is clearly no longer insulating people from the reality of exorbitant medical costs. With a greater percentage of every dollar earned going to pay for health care, consumers are being forced to make tough choices:

> On average, premiums for family coverage have risen by 62 percent since 2003 and now account for roughly 20 percent or more of the average American family's income, while deductibles have more than doubled. A general rule of thumb, as expressed in a recent report by the Altarum Institute, is that total medical cost (premiums and out-

of-pocket expenses) should not exceed 10 percent of family income. Above that limit, it is considered unaffordable, and the report highlights that 54 percent of middle-class families in the U.S. can no longer afford health insurance. That's a staggering number that has tripled in thirty years: in 1981 only 15 percent of middle-class families couldn't afford health insurance.[12]

Insurance costs are fast becoming the run-away train—completely out of control and waiting to derail. Schoen et al. extrapolated the future costs of health insurance based on the trend line and determined that "if insurance premiums for employer-sponsored health plans in each state continue to grow at the average annual rate for 2003–2011, the average premium for family coverage would rise to $24,700 by 2020, an increase of 65 percent from 2011."[13] The irrefutable bottom line is that employers and employees alike are being hammered and the future looks no brighter.

It should be noted that the average cost for family health insurance premiums "only" rose by 4 percent in 2013, according to the Kaiser Family Foundation. The same survey showed individual policies increased 5 percent. While the increases were small, they were multiples of the rates of inflation (1.1 percent) and wage increases (1.4 percent).[14]

A DIMINISHING BENEFIT

Faced with an increasingly unaffordable health benefits tab, employers worked aggressively to curtail costs. For some employers, cost reductions meant dropping coverage altogether; others retooled their benefit programs to make them far leaner. Care became more managed, as did pharmaceutical benefits, and employees bore an increasing responsibility to pay a portion of each health care dollar they spent.[15]

The first step for employers was to change the cost-sharing formula, which "resulted in an 80 percent increase in the annual costs of the employee's share for a single-person plan and a 74 percent increase in employee cost for a family plan from 2003 to 2011."[16]

The second step was to diminish the scope of benefits provided:

- "Almost three in four covered workers (73 percent) pay a copayment (a fixed dollar amount) for office visits with a primary care

physician, in addition to any general annual deductible their plan may have."[17]
- Workers also generally face similar cost sharing for prescription drugs, ER visits, outpatient services, and inpatient hospital care.[18]
- In 2006, on average, only 10 percent of workers participated in employer-sponsored plans with a deductible of $1,000 or more. By 2012, 34 percent faced such deductibles.[19]

The result of these actions is that "workers are thus paying more but getting less protective benefits."[20] But there's more to the story than merely reduced value to the employee.

The data suggests that dollars that might otherwise flow to employees in the form of salary increases or bonuses were allocated to paying the burgeoning health insurance premiums.[21] According to research conducted by the Kaiser Family Foundation and Health Research and Educational Trust, "since 2002, average premiums for family coverage have increased 97 percent. The growth in premiums has outpaced increases in both workers' wages (1.7 percent since 2011 and 33 percent since 2002) and inflation (2.3 percent since 2011 and 28 percent since 2002)."[22]

DROPPING COVERAGE

The most extreme method of controlling cost is for an employer to simply abdicate responsibility for the provision of health insurance. Evidence has shown that more employers have been dropping coverage, as "the likelihood of employment-based coverage declined from 64.4 percent in 1997 to 56.5 percent in 2010."[23]

Among these firms, there was a tremendous discrepancy in the levels of insurance offered based on company size. Larger firms seemed far more able to shoulder the costs than their smaller brethren: "Less than one half (45.3 percent) of people working in firms with fewer than twenty-five employees received health insurance benefits compared with 88.8 percent for people who worked for firms employing a thousand or more employees."[24]

THE UNINSURED AND UNDERINSURED

A recent survey shows that these trends resulted in a substantial number of Americans being either uninsured or underinsured at various
times:

- "As of 2010, estimates indicate eighty-one million adults under
  age sixty-five (44 percent of all adults) were either uninsured during the year or underinsured, up from sixty-one million in 2003."[25]
- "A 2011 survey by the CDC conducted in 2011 (National Health
  Interview Survey) showed 48.2 million Americans without insurance at the time of the survey—equal to 18.2 percent. Sixty-one
  point two percent were covered by private insurance."[26]
- "In the first nine months of 2012, 45.3 million persons of all ages
  (14.7 percent) were uninsured at the time of interview. 57.5 million (18.6 percent) had been uninsured for at least part of the year
  prior to interview, and 33.8 million (11.0 percent) had been uninsured for more than a year at the time of the interview."[27]

Who are these people? Some are youth who, convinced of their
invincibility, go without insurance. Some individuals have lost coverage
as a result of losing or changing jobs, and many are individuals who live
below the federal poverty line. Bleakly, the Kaiser Family Foundation
found that "among families with incomes below the federal poverty
level ($22,350 a year for a family of four in 2011), 40 percent are
uninsured."[28]

Certain demographic groups are also heavily affected by the lack of
insurance. The CDC's latest survey revealed that more than 25 percent
of the Hispanic population lacked health insurance and an even greater
percentage had gone without coverage during part of the previous
year.[29]

A lack of insurance results in more than unpayable medical bills. "A
review of the research literature over the past twenty-five years by
Hadley found that the uninsured receive fewer preventive and diagnostic services, tend to be more severely ill when diagnosed, and receive
less therapeutic care. He concluded that insurance coverage could reduce mortality by an estimated 4 to 25 percent, depending on the
condition."[30]

GROWING PUBLIC CONCERNS OVER COSTS

For consumers long isolated from the true costs of our health system, such expense is largely defined by what insurance does not pay, as corroborated by focus-group research conducted in 2012 by the Robert Wood Johnson Foundation. Participants defined those costs as out-of-pocket—be it for premiums, deductibles, copays, and so forth.[31]

Consumers were exquisitely aware of their costs. "Almost every person in every group could explain exactly—practically to the penny—what he/she spent on premiums, deductibles, and copays each month."[32] Their high levels of costs were forcing other changes among consumers, with participants saying that "they were cutting back on other areas of their lives in order to absorb rising health insurance premiums, copays, etc."[33]

The average consumer lacks the resources to manage this problem: "In 2012, more than two of five (41 percent) adults ages nineteen to sixty-four, or seventy-five million people, reported problems paying their medical bills or said they were paying off medical debt over time."[34]

THE ACA AND TRANSFORMATIONAL CHANGE

Soaring costs, the burdensome, punitive practices of insurers, and the growing pool of uninsured Americans have been churning in the cauldron of public opinion. The issues seem so vast as to be beyond the reasonable control of any group . . . other than the federal government.

In 2010, President Barack Obama accomplished what no other president before him had been able to do—he marshaled through a bill designed to bring unprecedented reform to the health insurance sector while broadening coverage to tens of millions of Americans. The law, known as the Affordable Care Act (ACA, also known as *Obamacare*), is more than two thousand pages in length and "includes several important coverage and delivery-system reforms designed to reduce cost growth and improve financial protection while also enhancing the quality of health care. The creation of state-based health insurance exchanges, introduction of new insurance-market rules and consumer protections, and expansion of state and federal oversight of industry practices provide a foundation for efforts to increase value in U.S. health insurance markets. Together, such provisions should begin to curb rising health insurance costs and make care and coverage more affordable."[35]

The passage of the law was followed by a tumultuous assault on its constitutionality, but it held up to the scrutiny. Due to its complexity, many of its key provisions phase in over an extended period. Arguably the most important provision, the creation and operation of state- and federally sponsored health insurance exchanges, occurred in 2014, with enrollment beginning in the fall of 2013. These exchanges are designed to provide affordable health insurance options devoid of onerous preexisting-condition clauses, lifetime limitations, or other sins of the past.

Beginning in 2014, some of the most critically important features of the ACA included the following:

- Guaranteed issue, in that "health plans must sell coverage to everyone, regardless of preexisting conditions, and can't charge more based on health or gender."[36]
- Health insurance exchanges (HIE), which function as central marketplaces where consumers can purchase insurance, exist at both the federal and state level. (ACA allows for both state-sponsored and federal exchanges.) The exchanges provide access to four levels of coverage, from plans with high out-of-pocket charges to more comprehensive plans. The vast majority of participants will enroll via the Web.
- Financial subsidies, which are being provided to improve the affordability of personal coverage. There are modest penalties for not obtaining coverage, either through one's employer, participation in an existing governmental plan, or the HIE. Employers also face modest penalties, which rise over time, for failing to provide coverage options.
- Increase in eligibility for participation in the Medicaid program, which is determined on a state-by-state basis.

The difficulty inherent in bringing this law to life was made readily apparent in July 2013 when it was announced that implementation of one of the most important provisions related to the provision of employer-sponsored health benefits would be delayed for one year: "The law passed in 2010 required employers with more than fifty employees working thirty or more hours a week to offer them suitable health coverage or pay a fine. Obama administration officials say they listened to businesses that complained they need to figure out how to comply with complicated new rules written since the plan became law."[37]

In August 2013 the *New York Times* published a story detailing another failure in the timely implementation of the ACA—one that could adversely affect consumers across the nation. According to author Robert Pear, "the limit on out-of-pocket costs, including deductibles and copayments, was not supposed to exceed $6,350 for an individual or $12,700 for a family. But under a little-noticed ruling, federal officials have granted a one-year grace period to some insurers, allowing them to set higher limits, or no limit at all on some costs, in 2014."[38] Numerous consumer-advocacy groups are jumping on the issue, exclaiming that the delay will prove to be very detrimental for chronically ill patients and others.

On October 1, 2013, the exchanges officially opened for business. Early enrollment of millions of diverse Americans was essential to the ultimate success of Obamacare. Unfortunately, a myriad of computer issues rendered the federal website, as well as many state websites, inaccessible or unusable by people trying to enroll. Ross Douthat, writing in the *New York Times*, bemoaned that "the online federal health care exchange, the heart of the Obamacare project, is such a rolling catastrophe that it may end up creating a major policy fiasco immediately rather than eventually."[39]

The president promised a rapid solution to the problem, which could dramatically alter the number of enrollees unless fixed in a timely fashion. Meanwhile, calls for the "head" of Health and Human Services, Secretary Kathleen Sebelius, echoed through the halls of Congress. Fortunately, the administration was able to remedy the problems, and enrollment began in earnest.

Despite its brutally awkward start, the ACA is already credited with some major accomplishments, having "already expanded coverage of young adults by allowing them to stay on their parents' plans until they turn twenty-six, outlawed lifetime limits on what insurance will cover, lowered the cost of drugs for seniors on Medicare, caused thirteen million consumers to get premium rebates totaling some $1.1 billion, and expanded access to free preventive care for patients of all ages."[40]

The impact on young adults has been immediate: "As a result of this early expansion, the percentage of young adults (ages nineteen to twenty-six) who were uninsured declined by nearly 4 percentage points over the past two years (from 31.4 percent to 27.7 percent), a dramatic departure from the steady increases over the early part of the decade."[41]

Other changes already in force include (1) the elimination of caps on annual and lifetime benefits for essential health care benefits—including such items as physician services, hospital or ambulatory services, medications, and disease management, and (2) access to an array of wellness services while prohibiting any associated charges or cost-sharing for these interventions. These services include a broad range of interventions, from screening mammography for women who qualify to vaccinations. Included services are based on guidelines from U.S. Preventative Services Task Force, Health Resources and Services Administration, and the CDC. A comprehensive list of covered services is available online.[42]

Coverage has and will continue to expand under ACA, but what about costs? It might be argued that by significantly improving access to the uninsured, the ACA opens up the funnel to allow more patients to flow into a dysfunctional, inefficient system. It may also raise costs, as some data indicates: "Although premiums are rising more slowly than they were before enactment of the recent reforms, private-insurance spending per person is projected to continue to grow more rapidly than incomes for the next decade."[43] Significantly expanded access to the health care system, I would argue, is the moral obligation of a nation as wealthy as ours. However, I would also argue that the tremendous dysfunction in the underlying system needs to be addressed with as much or more vigor first.

As Obamacare unfolds, other issues may materialize. One concern is the size of the networks offered to participants in some states. In an effort to offer price-competitive products, some insurance companies may drastically reduce the size of the networks by including only those providers willing to negotiate deep cost concessions. Such an approach will likely rule out most if not all academic medical centers. If enrollees then need the services of such centers and are forced to go out of network to obtain them, the costs to the enrollee may be unmanageable.

Elements of the Republican Party vowed to see the law repealed, though the probability of such an occurrence has become extraordinarily low with the passage of time. Even so, the level of impassioned rhetoric from the Republican Party included this comment by Representative John Fleming, MD, that appeared in the *New York Times*: "Obamacare is the most dangerous piece of legislation ever passed in Congress. It is the most existential threat to our economy, since the Great Depression."[44]

The greatest threat to the successful implementation of ACA lies in adverse risk selection, whereby only the sickest individuals enroll in plans while healthy young people remain on the sidelines, opting to pay a minor penalty in lieu of coverage. Since insurance companies rely on the ability to spread risks across a broad pool of applicants, such adverse risk selection could drive up the price of coverage. As costs escalate, in theory, adverse risk is intensified because only the sickest patients are willing to pay such premiums for coverage. The cycle of decreasing enrollment and escalating premiums makes the system unsustainable.

TODAY'S REALITY

Whether you champion or deride Obamacare, some incontrovertible facts about the statute remain:

- Our existing insurance system adds a tremendous administrative-cost burden to the already exorbitant national health care bill.
- The insurance industry, as well as the federal government, have done pathetically little to curb the outrageous pricing of health care services—which the ACA is unlikely to change.
- There has been tremendous push back on state-sponsored health exchanges, as well as expansion of the Medicaid program.
- Millions of Americans will still be without coverage—including a disproportionate share of impoverished Americans.
- "While all states may eventually choose to participate in the expansion [of the Medicaid program] over the next decade, poor families in many states will continue to be at risk of going without health insurance even after the Affordable Care Act goes into full effect in 2014."[45]

There are also innumerable, unanswered questions, beginning with figuring out where all the providers needed to treat the swelling ranks of Medicaid enrollees will come from . . . particularly in an era of increasing physician shortages.

THE GRAVY TRAIN CONTINUES FOR INSURERS

The ACA is having an impact on insurers' bottom lines—just not the intended impact of controlling costs. Frier found that "insurance companies spent millions of dollars trying to defeat the U.S. health care overhaul, saying it would raise costs and disrupt coverage. Instead, profit margins at the companies widened to levels not seen since before the recession, a Bloomberg Government study shows."[46] In fact, she goes on to point out that "insurers led by WellPoint Inc. (WLP), the biggest [insurer] by membership, recorded their highest combined quarterly net incomes of the past decade after the law was signed in 2010."[47]

There appears to be more evidence that insurers have already learned how to game the system: "According to an analysis by HCAN, Wall Street–run health insurance companies took $7 billion in profits in the first half of 2011 by charging more and spending much less on patient care. Combined profits for UnitedHealth Group, Inc.; WellPoint, Inc.; Aetna, Inc.; Cigna Corp; and Humana, Inc.—which cover one-third of the U.S. population—surged toward expected profits of $14 billion for 2011, a record. Through the economic recession and its aftermath from 2008 to 2010, combined profits for the five companies increased by 51 percent."[48]

What are insurance companies doing with all this money? Like pharma, they appear to be paying it out in exorbitant salaries to their executives. Take Stephen Hemsley, CEO of UnitedHealth Group, for example. According to *Forbes*'s 2012 survey of top CEO compensation, Hemsley's five-year compensation was pegged at $169.3 million.[49] With forty-five million Americans without health care coverage, this type of compensation raises interesting ethical questions.

Afraid that the gravy train may be slowing, there's speculation that insurers are seeking new ways to maintain price escalation on premiums and hence profitability. One method might be to buddy up with health care actuaries to inflate the estimated costs of coverage, thus justifying larger rate increases in the future. Some observers, including Minnesota senator Al Franken, already accuse actuaries of being joined at the hip with insurers.[50]

In March 2013 the Society of Actuaries published a study "predicting that, thanks to sicker patients joining the coverage pool, medical claims per member will rise 32 percent in the individual plans expected to dominate the ACA exchanges next year."[51] The report went on to state that cost increases will be as high as 80 percent in some markets.[52]

The ACA brings needed but highly incremental reforms to health care. Most importantly, it appears to do little to change the underlying cost structure its greatest problem.

WHAT YOU CAN DO TO PROTECT YOUR HEALTH

The type and level of health care coverage you and your family enjoy determine the financial impact you feel every time you interact with the health care system. If you are among the tens of millions of Americans who are uninsured, the ACA may bring you relief long before you are hit with unmanageable medical expenses. If your insurance affords you robust benefits and your share of the expenses is low to moderate, the pinch will be minor. If you have a high-deductible plan with major cost sharing, the pain will be commensurately greater but somewhat offset by lower premium costs.

A more difficult challenge is determining whether you are underinsured. That's why it is essential that you understand the provisions of your policy and what health care expenses are included, excluded, or shared. Some plans have extremely low premiums and correspondingly low benefits.

Even with very good coverage, you may encounter problems, the most onerous of which for many patients is a denial. An insurance denial occurs when your insurance company refuses to pay for treatment. The reasons are many, but the two most common are (1) because an error was made somewhere along the line causing either the wrong treatment or wrong diagnosis to appear on a preapproval request or claim and (2) because the insurer denied coverage by refuting the appropriateness of the treatment method. While one can be remedied with relative ease, the other is more difficult.

Insurance companies are governed by rules of engagement that broadly define what treatments are permissible for given conditions. As a general rule of thumb, insurers may exclude modalities deemed experimental or lacking in scientific evidence that supports their comparative efficacy over other treatments. Rarely questioned are treatments that have become "standards of care" within the profession.

An example is the use of the drug Avastin to treat cancer patients. This tremendously expensive drug has proven efficacy in the treatment of some colon cancers. Because of these results, many doctors and their patients wanted to use it for other cancers, such as breast, where there was no scientific proof of efficacy. Insurers denied coverage in many cases and were publicly chastised for doing so. When the evidence did mount, it was against the use of Avastin for breast cancer, because it was ineffective—vindicating the stance of insurers: "On November 18, 2011, Food and Drug Administration commissioner Margaret Hamburg revoked the agency's accelerated approval of the breast cancer indication for bevacizumab (Avastin®, made by Genentech). Bevacizumab used for metastatic breast cancer has not been shown to provide a benefit, in terms of delay in the growth of tumors, that would justify its serious and potentially life-threatening risks. Nor is there evidence that use of bevacizumab will either help women with breast cancer live longer or improve their quality of life."[53]

Your insurance company should provide you with a document explaining their denial, as well as any supportive documentation required to further illuminate their rationale. Your job is to seek to understand both your physician's perspective when ordering the treatment as well as the insurer's perspective when denying it. There may be validity to each perspective. If your physician deems the treatment essential and has no discernible economic conflicts of interest that might predispose recommendation of a particular modality of care, then you need to fight for your rights. Your physician alone can build an argument using current research and clinical data to support a treatment recommendation, and so your physician must be your advocate. You can also do your own research within the clinical literature, though most laypeople find the reading to be tough sledding.

If your appeal to the insurance company is subsequently denied, the door still has not permanently shut on your case. Most states have some form of health insurance advocacy department for consumers—usually organized under the insurance commissioner. In my home state of Kansas, it is the Kansas Insurance Departments Consumer Assistance Division. These organizations can help you understand your options and provide guidance on next steps.

There are also important, new protections offered under the ACA:

> Before the Affordable Care Act was passed, people's rights to appeal decisions made by their health plans varied depending on where they lived, what type of health plan they had, and whether they bought insurance themselves or got it through their job. In some states, when people disagreed with their health plan's decision, they could appeal that decision outside of their health plan, and in other states they had no appeal rights.
>
> Under the Affordable Care Act, if you disagree with your plan's refusal to pay for care, the plan will have to review its decision. And if you still are not satisfied, you will have the right to appeal that decision to an independent reviewer who is outside of the health plan.[54]

If you are covered by a governmental plan, such as Medicare, a separate process exists for appealing denials. According to the Medicare website, you can file appeals regarding

- a request for a health care service, supply, item, or prescription drug that you think you should be able to get;
- a request for payment of a health care service, supply, item, or prescription drug you already got;
- a request to change the amount you must pay for a health care service, supply, item, or prescription drug; and
- your Medicare health plan or your Medicare drug plan, if the latter stops providing or paying for all or part of a health care service, supply, item, or prescription drug you think you still need.[55]

This same site will walk you through the five levels of appeal provided by the federal government. Medicaid denials go through their own process, with some degree of variance among states. One online source that may be helpful in this regard is NOLO's page on how to appeal a denial of Medicaid.[56]

If you are unable to afford a treatment that your physician feels is essential because of either lack of coverage or denial, it may be possible for your physician to advocate to the hospital to work with you to make the needed treatment affordable without running afoul of any regulatory restrictions. Great care needs to be exercised whenever modifying fees for treatment—particularly when governmental payers are involved.

It should also be noted that many pharmaceutical manufacturers and device companies have provisions for helping the medically indigent gain access to their products. You may wish to research this topic and then ask for your physician's advocacy as appropriate.

You may also wish to avail yourself of an emerging new profession, the private health care advocate, who may play a role in helping you overcome obstacles with your insurance companies. Advocates vary in terms of their core competencies and services but often help their clients determine

- whether they are getting the appropriate standard of care based on their diagnoses;
- whether they are utilizing the best, available, and affordable resources;
- whether their medical bills are correct; and
- how to manage any issues, including denials, with insurance companies.

Keep in mind that there are no criteria for assessing an advocate's competency, nor are their licensure requirements or recognized certifications. In other words, caveat emptor. With that admonishment, an advocate may still be an invaluable asset as you seek to resolve difficult issues.

A final way to improve your health is by taking advantage of the many incentives now being offered by employers and insurance companies for participation in wellness programs. Since employers and insurers are largely footing the bill for your care, they want you to stay well; hence they are willing to incentivize the right behavior in the hope that you make meaningful lifestyle changes.

MYTH 10
"WHEN ALL ELSE FAILS, AT LEAST THE SYSTEM WILL ALLOW ME TO DIE WITH DIGNITY"

Every family has its rituals, and one of ours was Sunday-night dinner. It was a time to share news, to talk about our hopes or dreams, to simply relish time spent together. Sunday, May 20, 2001, was no exception. I went home after dinner, counting my blessings—so grateful to have my parents, despite their advancing ages.

On Monday, a call from my mother changed my world. My father had slept in, which, despite being eighty-six years old, was not his habit. When she went to rouse him, there was no response. He seemed to be breathing okay but was completely unresponsive. That's when I got the frantic call.

So began our final odyssey with my father . . . a trip that would take us into the deepest realms of the health care system.

Eight minutes after calling 911, EMS paramedics were onsite preparing my father to be transported to a nearby emergency room. Upon arrival at the hospital, the frenetic pace of the first responders was replaced by long hours of waiting as my father slowly moved from the ER to the ICU. There, a team of specialists went to work seeking to identify the underlying cause of his condition.

My father remained in a coma throughout that week, during which time our family maintained a vigil at the ICU. The waiting room, our temporary home, was bathed in the green sterile glow of fluorescent lights. It was a spaced shared with other families in crisis. Its eerie quiet was punctuated only by breathless sobs as bad news was delivered to loved ones. Whenever possible, we escaped to be at my father's bedside, though watching the life slowly ebb from this once-strong man was so painful.

Toward the end of the week, the doctors informed us that an underlying blood disease had transformed into a fulminating type of leukemia, from which my father would not recover. We were told that the merciful thing to do would be to let him go. When I asked for more information on which to make such a difficult decision, my father's oncologist turned away from me and directed her response to my brother, a physician. She seemed annoyed that I would not blindly accept what had been recommended and cloaked her response in impenetrable medical jargon.

I again asked a series of questions—including whether my father was aware of his surroundings. A different physician addressed me directly and provided assurance that my father had no awareness and promised that he would quietly pass when we removed life support. After a family conference, we agreed to take him off the respirator.

As my father's lungs labored for breath, he raised his arms up over his head and let them drop. I shot a sharp look at the ICU physician, who said that it was nothing more than a muscular reaction. My father repeated this motion several times before giving up. It was no simple twitch . . . it was more of a plea not to give up. His instructions to us had always been, "Do everything in your power to keep me alive." He was a fighter with an indomitable spirit. I will always feel that we let him down.

I hugged him for a last time, told him how much I loved him and would miss him, and said goodbye. I promised my nearly atheistic father that he was in for a beautiful surprise at what lay ahead of him.

After we had said our collective goodbyes in the bustling ICU, my brother and I took my mother's arms and walked her out. Her inseparable partner for sixty-one years was gone.

My brother and I feared that it would not be long before we lost our mother. Life without her soul mate would simply be too much to endure. But thankfully she proved us wrong and lived another six years.

My mother's death could not have been more different and opened my eyes to what Dr. Ira Byock refers to as "dying well."

As my mother approached her eighty-eighth birthday, it was clear that she was growing weary of life without my father, as well as contending with an increasingly long list of infirmities. Due to a series of falls, she was tended by caregivers in her home twenty-four hours a day, as arranged by my brother and I. This, too, she tired of but accepted as a condition of maintaining some level of independent living.

Despite the careful eyes of her caregivers, she nonetheless fell again, this time breaking her knee. She was briefly hospitalized, during which time she was evaluated by an orthopedic surgeon. After viewing her X-rays, he recommended an immediate operation to pin the broken bone.

I asked if he was aware of my mother's staggeringly high blood pressure and poorly controlled diabetes. He said yes. I asked if these conditions would substantially increase the risk of surgery. He grudgingly said yes. Finally, I asked what would happen if we did nothing other than bed rest. He indicated it would probably take an additional two to three weeks for her bones to heal.

It was stunning to me that the surgeon was willing to trade off a couple of meager weeks of bed rest for a significant risk of surgical complications or death. My mother and I agreed that it was time to leave the hospital and go home. I informed the orthopedic surgeon that there would be no operation.

I'm not sure exactly when it happened during my mother's convalescence, but at some point she decided it was time to let go. The fight was over, and she was ready to join my father. So she simply stopped eating.

I sat on the edge of her bed and asked if she knew what she was doing. She told me that she had been graced with a glorious life and it was time to say goodbye. Her knee was mending. That was not the issue. My mother had watched as more and more elements of her life lay beyond her control. Through a simple, passive action, she could regain control and direct the remaining course of her days on earth.

It would take many weeks for my mother to pass. We brought in hospice, which helped us maintain her comfort and manage any pain or anxiety. Though painful to anticipate her loss, we nonetheless managed to savor every moment with my mother.

In the last few weeks, she became very confused and fatigued. Lucid moments seemed to be forever gone. I knew that death was near as I arrived early one morning to check on her. I was prepared to see the progressive and inevitable decline that had marked each of the past few *days. But instead I found my mother sitting in bed fully awake. She said, "John, honey, come here; I want to talk with you."*

Something incredibly powerful and unexplainable was happening. My mother was completely lucid and focused. It was as though her age and infirmity had been momentarily erased. She spoke with exacting clarity—wanting to ensure that I took in every measure of love and wisdom being doled out.

She said, "Remember how much your father and I treasured you. Always carry our love with you. And know that we will be looking down upon you. . . . We will always be with you."

I told her I loved her and reassured her that she wasn't going anywhere quite yet. . . . It wasn't her time. But my mother knew differently. She told me she had to rest. That was the last time I spoke with my mother. She passed away the next evening with my wife and me at her side. I held her hand as her body took its final breath. There was a peace in life's finality.

I had once asked Elisabeth Kübler-Ross what happens at the moment we die. "It's like a cocoon," she told me. "When a butterfly is ready, the cocoon opens up, and out comes a butterfly."

That's how I choose to remember my mother's passing—like a cocoon opening to let a beautiful butterfly soar.

I witnessed two parents die under very different circumstances: one confined to an ICU and tethered to a ventilator, the other lying peacefully in bed at home surrounded by loved ones. The experiences could not have been more different, and the lessons learned will stay with me forever.

DEATH IS NOT THE ENEMY

Whether driven by cultural narcissism or some unique feature of our genetic makeup, most Americans are undeniably unaccepting of the inevitability of death. "Let's face it," George Lundberg put it succinctly, "no one wants to die, but everyone must. Despite this overwhelming reality, we continue to chase the illusion of life everlasting."[1]

This lack of understanding and avoidance of the reality of death come at a price. Without discussion, our fears, hopes, and final wishes go unattended. As Otis Brawley observed, "We cannot accept that death will come, and thus we cannot make a plan, talk reasonably about it, work our way to understanding, to the basic part of our humanity."[2]

Yet as Lundberg and others have pointed out, death is not the enemy. "The real enemies of medicine are premature death, disease, disability, pain, human suffering."[3] Kübler-Ross would add "peace and dignity" to the list of casualties in our battle with death, warning that "we would think that our great emancipation, our knowledge of science and of man, has given us better ways and means to prepare ourselves and our families for this inevitable happening. Instead the days are gone when a man was allowed to die in peace and dignity in his own house."[4]

THE ROAD NOT TAKEN

> Two roads diverged in a wood, and I—
> I took the one less traveled by,
> And that has made all the difference.[5]

Nowhere do Robert Frost's words ring more true than when facing end-of-life decisions. One path, if pursued to the end, leads to a medicalized death. Along the way, every tool, technology, and craft of the trade is used by physicians to preserve life. It often begins in the ER and ends in the ICU, as it did with my father.

This is the path most chosen, as revealed by a survey of more than eight thousand patients who had visited an ER—15 percent of whom would die within six months of the visit.[6] The ER is the trailhead of a path leading to a death that is, at best, "lonely and impersonal."[7]

Others cast dying in a far more dismal light. Ira Byock, MD, past president of the American Society for Palliative and Hospice Medicine, recalled darkly that "if death on the wards was macabre, in the ER it was ghastly. In the hands of the medical system, even passings that should have been peaceful turned gruesome."[8]

Many patients travel beyond the ER, as "hospitalization also was common following an emergency department visit toward the end of life. Among the 2,157 participants who visited the emergency department in the last month of life, 77 percent were subsequently hospitalized. Of those who were hospitalized, 39 percent were admitted to an intensive care unit, and 68 percent died in the hospital."[9]

Some people are fighters. They don't want to give up. They want the full capabilities of the health care system enlisted in their battle for life, up until the last minute. Others enter the system as fighters but learn the hard way that "a sophisticated hospital is the last place you want to be when terminally ill. Once you're in the hospital setting, you're trapped. The staff owns you, and they do all those terrible things they have been trained to do to prolong life, no matter how artificially or how hopelessly."[10]

How does this happen? Part of the answer lies in the culture of medicine that abhors giving up the battle for life. Part also lies in the depersonalization of care that Kübler-Ross alluded to: "All too often today's decisions about prolonging life through aggressive application of high technology are made by specialists who know their patients only as a 'case.'"[11]

When the probable benefits of the care are vastly superseded by the pain, suffering, and costs of that care, it is labeled *futile care*. Lundberg notes it as a "particularly onerous deviation from quality standards" and condemns "the practice of subjecting terminally ill patients to painful, costly, debilitating treatments that offer little or no hope of any meaningful recovery." He goes on to add that

> No accurate assessments of the dollar cost of futile care are available, but it surely adds up to many billions, raked in by hospitals and physicians. The emotional cost of futile care has been felt by millions of patients and families. Time and time again, people say they do not want to end their lives hooked up to respirators, IVs, and monitoring devices, but when in the final stages of a terminal illness they are admitted to a sophisticated medical center, that is precisely how they end their lives. Futile care, a contradiction in terms, is the most distressing example of the search for cure taking precedence over the need for true care.[12]

The patient who has chosen this path "may cry for rest, peace, and dignity, but he will get infusions, transfusions, a heart machine, or tracheotomy if necessary."[13] Or, as Lundberg grimly summed it up, "when patients near death, we often disregard their express wishes, as recorded in living wills, instead pummeling, prodding, infusing, and respirating them until what remains no longer resembles the parent, spouse, or sibling the family once knew."[14]

THERE IS ANOTHER PATH AT THE END OF LIFE

Rather than being driven by technology, the other path at the end of life is driven by the heart. It begins with an acceptance of the patient's condition and a desire to make this final stage of life meaningful. It requires a committed team of caregivers whose focus is on making the patient comfortable, pain free, and able to bring closure to their lives. In America, it is the path less traveled.

This path is predicated on the belief that "if a patient is allowed to terminate his life in the familiar and beloved environment, it requires less adjustment for him. His own family knows him well enough to replace a sedative with a glass of his favorite wine, or the smell of a home-cooked soup may give him the appetite to sip a few spoons of fluid, which, I think is still more enjoyable than an infusion."[15] It is a gift not only to the patient but to all who are allowed to participate in the dying process.

In his book *Dying Well* Dr. Ira Byock recounts the story of his father's death and the lessons learned:

> On Friday, forty-eight hours after his decision to die in our home, Dad slipped beyond responding. We still talked softly to him as we moistened his lips, bathed him, or changed his pajamas. At this point our "I love you, Dad," or Mom's "I love you, Seymour," needed no response. We just needed to say them.
>
> This time felt sacred, but not in the way that scripture, liturgy, or chants are sacred. There was a luminous—or numinous—quality to the moment. A great man was passing. So much was being lost, but, oh, what a treasure he was. What a privilege to have known him, to have loved and been loved by him and to have been raised by him.[16]

The process of watching his father die peacefully and with dignity was transformative for Byock:

> I had grown accustomed to seeing death through medical eyes; my father's cancer forced me to experience terminal illness from the vantage point of a patient's family. Furthermore, through my father's eyes, I glimpsed dying from the point of view of a person living in the shadow of death. Dad's dying was certainly not the happiest time in our family's life, but as a family we had never been more intimate, more open, or more openly loving. His illness allowed us, I could say

forced us, to talk about the things that mattered: family, our relationships with one another, our shared past, and the unknown future. We
reminisced about good times and bad, we cried, and we laughed. We
apologized for a host of transgressions, and we granted, and were
granted, forgiveness. Through Dad's illness and in his dying we all
grew individually and together.[17]

This path, which can be so virtuous, requires a skilled guide—physicians and nurses who understand and embrace the concept of dying
well. These lessons are learned in the trenches, watching as patients
and their families go through end-of-life experiences. But it takes more
than passive observation. It requires a physician to be open and aware
enough to understand the delicate balance between supporting life and
supporting a patient's wishes as they approach death. It is the priestly
side of medicine that allows the physician to relinquish the secular in
favor of the sacred.

WHAT'S MISSING FROM MEDICAL SCHOOL: LESSONS IN DYING

What do we, as a society, ultimately expect from our physicians relative
to end-of-life care? As Kübler-Ross put it, "we have to ask ourselves
whether medicine is to remain a humanitarian and respected profession
or a new but depersonalized science in the service of prolonging life
rather than diminishing human suffering."[18] In the decades since she
wrote these words, we've moved far down the scientific path.

A course correction will require a change in medical education.
Medical students will need to understand the artful management of the
dying, just as they understand how to support life. "We need to train
physicians not only to fight for life but also to accept the end of life,"
insists Lundberg. "We have to train physicians to be humane caregivers,
to listen to their patients, and to ease their way to death."[19]

Aspiring physicians will also need a lesson in hope. Every doctor
learns of the five stages of death and dying identified by Kübler-Ross.
When asked what she would add to her work on death and dying, she
responded, "I would add a chapter on hope. At the beginning, when
people are diagnosed with cancer, their hope is always for a cure or at
least for the prolongation of life. When they go through the stages, if

they reach acceptance, you can diagnose it from the outside by asking them what is their hope. It never has anything to do with a cure or the prolongation of life. It has to do with things like acceptance by God in his garden. The quality of hope changes depending upon what stage the patient is in."[20]

Changes to medical education will work only if there is a fundamental change in the culture of medicine. In the current culture "physicians are very upset if you suggest sending a patient to hospice, for it means they have failed as physicians."[21] These physicians want to employ ever-more-powerful medications or other interventions in the slim hope of changing the patient's condition. In such cases, technology becomes a tool of last resort with little utility, when patients still have profound needs from their caregivers. But "what they need is more attentive care," says Lundberg. "They need physicians who will listen to them and their families and who will talk about the nature of their terminal illnesses. In some clearly defined situations, they need doctors who will help them die."[22] It should be noted that the intent is not to promote that physicians actively intervene in or accelerate the dying process but, rather, that they understand and respect a patient's wishes and then collaborate with the patient and the family to achieve a "good" death.

THE ECONOMIC COST OF DYING IN AMERICA

The culture of medicine and its attitude toward death causes not only physical and mental suffering but financial angst as well. Most of us are acquainted with statistics that demonstrate how dramatically spending increases toward the end of life: "No one seems to argue with the estimate that about 24 percent of Medicare spending and about 15 percent of all health spending is incurred in the last year of a patient's life."[23]

As our doctors wage an unwinnable battle, more and more resources are consumed. The patient undergoes more interventions but fares no better, as demonstrated in a study by Fisher et al. published in 2003 by the *Annals of Internal Medicine*:

> Fisher and his colleagues looked at the costs and health results of
> end-of-life care for people with hip fractures, colorectal cancer, or

acute myocardial infarctions. He found patients in the study's high-est-spending areas get approximately 60 percent more health care—for minor procedures, physician visits, tests, and hospital and special-ist use—but experienced no better health outcomes, satisfaction with their care, or superior functioning as a result. In fact, the extra care increased mortality by 2 to 5 percent—probably from patients being subjected to the dangers inherent in being hospitalized such as in-creased risk of infection, Wennberg, Fisher, and others have theor-ized.[24]

The actual costs per patient are quite high and quite variable across geographies, which comes as no surprise based on the geographic varia-tions in health care delivery. The Dartmouth Atlas examined the costs associated with end-of-life care by looking at Medicare expenditures at the end of life. The researchers found that "Medicare spent $43,500 on hospitalized patients in the last two years of life in Los Angeles, the fifth-highest regional tab in the country. In contrast, it spent 20 percent less on patients in San Francisco, 36 percent less in San Diego, and 67 percent less in Sacramento."[25]

GETTING IT RIGHT: ADVANCING PALLIATIVE CARE

There is one field of medicine that is trying to get it right: palliative care, which "focuses on the prevention and relief of suffering through the meticulous management of symptoms from the early through the final stages of an illness; it attends closely to the emotional, spiritual, and practical needs of patients and those close to them."[26]

Palliative-medicine specialists are experts in the management of pain. They know that pain, even the seemingly intractable pain of a terminal illness, can usually be contained. They also know that patients continue to suffer needlessly despite this fact. Byock boldly asserts that "physical pain among the terminally ill exists because doctors lack the will, not the way. With strong resolve from patient and doctor, relief of *physical* suffering is *always* possible."[27]

The key is getting patients under the care of palliative specialists—and doing so in a timely manner. There are several limiting factors, however, at play here: (1) There are a finite number of palliative-care specialists in practice, though the number is growing, (2) many physicians may be reluctant to hand off responsibility to such a physician—seeing it as either an abdication of their responsibility to the patient or a failure of treatment—and (3) the patient may be resistant, believing that it signifies "giving up" before they are ready to do so. In reality, patients may be under the supervision of a palliative physician for years.

As Smith et al. note, "early enrollment in outpatient palliative-care services has shown great promise in improving the quality of life for patients with serious illness, but access to these services remains limited."[28]

Hospitals are also beginning to establish inpatient palliative-care units for those patients who are noncurative but nonetheless require significant symptom management. These units are less acute (and less expensive) than intensive care units but offer more clinical support than can be delivered via homecare or on an outpatient basis. As such, these units appear to fill an important and growing niche.[29]

LESSONS FROM THE EDGE

I would be remiss not to acknowledge a less-scientific but nonetheless fascinating and popular area of investigation related to the end of life: the near-death experience. The body of literature surrounding near-death experiences, or NDEs, has grown dramatically in recent years. These case studies and personal anecdotes focus on patients who were momentarily clinically dead and subsequently resuscitated. They are recounted by physicians, nurses, and other caregivers, as well as the patients themselves.

The earliest such case was reported by Elisabeth Kübler-Ross, which she recounted to me in an interview at her home in 1997:

> My first insight came from a patient named Mrs. Schwartz. She told me how she died in a hospital in Indiana. She said her soul floated out of her body. She heard every word that people said. She described the resuscitation team in detail. She even repeated a joke of one of the young residents, who was very apprehensive when she didn't seem to respond. She repeated the whole joke—heard at a time when she had no vital signs. That was our first near-death experience ever recorded. Eighty medical and theology students heard her tell this story.

> My students attacked me for listening to this woman. They said it
> was an illusion or a hallucination. I told them that if I were to blow a
> dog whistle in the room, none of them would hear it. That doesn't
> mean that the sound does not exist.[30]

Kübler-Ross's students may have chastised her for telling such an unorthodox tale, but it did not dissuade her from devoting her life to reporting on thousands of case studies of the dying, many of which included NDEs.

Regardless of the source, the most striking thing about NDE literature is the commonality of experience among patients during the time of death. Most patients report an initial sense of being *out of body*. They report hovering above their body—watching the heroic interventions being performed in the hope of bringing them back to life. There is no pain, nor fear, no desire to return to the body. These patients are often able to recount specific events or the content of conversations that they could not possibly be privy to while deeply anesthetized. Some patients describe the unpleasant sensation of suddenly being "sucked back into their bodies"—which is uniformly described as jarring, painful, and unwelcome.

For others, the journey continues as their clinical death grows longer in duration. They may find themselves traveling at great speed through a tunnel of brilliant light. The light is often imbued with the divine characteristic of unconditional love. People speak of being "bathed in the light of unconditional love." Depending on their faiths, patients may describe the light as God.

At some point, they reach the end of the tunnel. There is more variance in what happens next. For some, it is a jolting return to the body. For others, there is a conversation with deceased relatives—during which they may be told that it is not their "time" and thus they must return to their bodies. Some patients experience what is referred to as a "life review," in which they see the entirety of their lives in what feels like mere seconds. Rarely are there negative associations, other than when the victims must return to their bodies, leaving the comfort of the light behind.

Adults and children often experience many of the same phenomena, including the tunnel of light and the extraordinary sense of love and well-being. They may experience relatives, religious figures, or what they describe as "angels."

Are these experiences real, or are they the random firing of neurons within an oxygen-starved brain as it begins its finally shut down? It's impossible to know. None of us can answer that question until we cross over . . . or don't. In the interim, based on the sheer volume and continuity of reports, I will choose to accept the reality of NDEs as res ipsa loquitur—the experience speaks for itself.

Let me close this important chapter with succinct and cogent advice from Ira Byock. "When the human dimension of dying is nurtured," he writes, "for many the transition from life can become as profound, intimate, and precious as the miracle of birth."[31]

WHAT YOU CAN DO TO PROTECT YOUR HEALTH

The first step is to define what you want to happen at the end of your life. Rather than leaving things to chance and the whims of an overly aggressive health care system, it would be wise to articulate your wishes about how the final stage of your life will be managed.

Do you want every possible medical intervention performed, regardless of the probability of extending your life, or do you want, at some point, for all but supportive care to be terminated? Such decisions are not easily made and require both soul searching and considerable discussion with your loved ones and physician. When you do come to peace with a decision, it needs to be formally codified in the form of advanced directives.

Advanced directives generally take one of three forms: (1) a living will, (2) a durable power of attorney for health care matters (DPOA-HC), or (3) a do-not-resuscitate order (DNR). It is important to understand the limitations of each directive, which may vary from state to state.

A living will provides your loved ones and caregivers with general instructions about how you wish to be treated in the event you are unable to participate in treatment decisions. It is a kind of instruction book on your care during the end of your life, and it is written in a very broad fashion. It may, however, not be legally binding.

The DPOA-HC, on the other hand, is a legally binding agreement between you and your advocate (someone whom you trust implicitly to act in your best interest and in tandem with your wishes). The DPOA-

HC takes effect when it is determined by medical professions that you are no longer able to participate in decisions regarding your health care. Your advocate then assumes responsibility for directing your care, including making such decisions as

- determining whether or not to continue medical care;
- electing to withhold food and water in cases of terminal illness (or unrecoverable brain injury), including the withdrawal of feeding tubes; and
- determining whether you will die in the hospital, a nursing home, or at home.

Numerous organizations publish samples of DPOAs on their websites, including the University of Michigan Health Care System. Following is one brief excerpt from their well-constructed document.

Life Support

Some people want to decide what types of life-support treatments and medicines they get from doctors to help them live longer when they are sick. Read through all six choices, and initial the one that best fits what you want or do not want to happen if you are very sick.

_____ I want doctors to do everything they think might help me. Even if I am very sick and I have little hope of getting better, I want them to keep me alive for as long as they can.

_____ I want doctors to do everything they think might help me, but, if I am very sick and I have little hope of getting better, I do NOT want to stay on life support.

_____ I want doctors to do everything they think might help me, but (initial all that apply):

_____ I don't want doctors to restart my heart if it stops by using CPR.

_____ I don't want a ventilator to pump air into my lungs if I cannot breathe on my own.

_____ I don't want a dialysis machine to clean my blood if my kidneys stop working.

_____ I don't want a feeding tube if I can't swallow.

_____ I don't want a blood transfusion if I need blood.

_____ I don't want any life support treatment.

_____ I want my Patient Advocate to decide for me.

_____ I am not sure.
_____ Other[32]

A DNR indicates that a patient whose heart stops or who stops breathing is not to be resuscitated. A DNR clearly applies only to terminal patients who desire a "natural" death. There is significant variation in the degree to which DNRs may be applied in various settings based on prevailing state laws. Furthermore, EMS personnel may be required to resuscitate even in the presence of a DNR if called to an emergency.

A DNR can be a merciful order to put in place when there is no hope of recovery, but it always requires significant deliberation.

It is important to note that all three advanced directives can be changed at will by the patient while the patient is of sound mind.

Advanced directives are not always honored for a broad array of reasons: Sometimes providers are unaware of their existence; at other times they choose to disregard them because no one is actively advocating for the patient. Additionally, some faith-based organizations may deem a patient's advance directives to be in direct conflict with their stated values and policies. Even state laws may intrude on the ability to honor a patient's advanced directives. For these reasons, it is extremely important that you have confidence in your physician's willingness to honor your wishes, as well as your family's support for your advanced directives.

That's why you may also wish to consider a fourth directive that was developed two decades ago in Oregon. Physician orders for life-sustaining treatment (POLST) were designed to ensure a high level of compliance with patients' final wishes. "POLST encourages communication between providers and patients, enabling patients to make more informed decisions. POLST guides patients through the risks and benefits of medical treatment pertinent to their own medical situation so that they can request or refuse certain measures."[33]

According to O'Malley and Zweibel, "among patients with a completed POLST, treatment preferences were respected 98 percent of the time and no one received unwanted resuscitation, intensive care, or breathing or feeding tubes."[34]

Finally, it is important to have a clear understanding of the degree to which your medical condition will likely impair the quality of your life over time. A woman diagnosed with Stage IV, terminal breast cancer may nonetheless live a number of years with a relatively high quality of life. For such an individual, among the most important aspects of care will be astute pain management as her condition gradually deteriorates.

Conversely, a person diagnosed with a devastating neurological condition, such as amyotrophic lateral sclerosis will likely see their quality of life decline precipitously—potentially hastening their decision regarding the appropriateness of life-sustaining interventions.

Few of us want to give up and surrender our precious lives. But even fewer of us want to suffer unnecessarily.

EPILOGUE

My objective has been to open your eyes to the profound need for transformational change within health care. I've also sought to make it crystal clear that a single piece of legislation, such as Obamacare, is not the answer to health care's problems. In truth, there is no panacea for the profound woes of American medicine.

Nonetheless, with the information provided in this book, you should be in a better position to maintain your health while improving the care you receive from the system. It won't be easy to discern the best decisions at critical moments, but at least you are no longer flying blind.

There's something more, though, that I hope will happen as a result of reading this book.

It is my fervent hope that some of you will choose to "act up" and not accept the status quo of our health care system. Ordinary citizens can exert extraordinary power to change or transform organizations that are failing to live up to societal values. When the efforts of citizens are combined with efforts from transformational leaders within the industry who are equally desperate for change, the resulting synergy can rapidly catalyze unprecedented transformation.

I believe that despite its "bad apples," there are plenty of physicians, hospital administrators, and pharmaceutical executives who believe that things need to change—and change now. I also believe that they will respond to the voice of the consumer once it reaches an appropriate crescendo.

If you agree, let me provide a few thoughts about your next steps. First, you need to codify your beliefs regarding the changes you feel are essential within health care. It will serve to anchor you as you begin to advocate for change. Try to answer the following questions for yourself:

- What would define professionalism for me relative to my physicians?
- What level of error should I be willing to tolerate from the health care system? Is it reasonable to expect, for instance, that I will not suffer from a hospital-induced injury or illness during a hospitalization?
- What should be done to protect me from incompetent or compromised physicians or other providers?
- Can I reasonably expect that my treatment options will be clearly and accurately explained to me and that I will be provided with scientifically accurate data on which to base my decisions?
- Should I be able to discern the true cost of my care regardless of who is paying for it?
- Should I be able to differentiate between the quality of various providers based on quantitative-outcomes data and patient-satisfaction data?
- Is it reasonable for me to know whether my physician has a vested interest or profits financially through the provision of certain treatments?
- Should I expect that research underlying pharmaceutical claims will adhere to the highest research standards and that there will be tremendously damaging fines for abusive practices by the pharmaceutical industry?
- Can I trust that my attitudes and views toward end-of-life care will be respected?
- Can I hope to be kept relatively pain free, if at all possible, during the terminal stages of illness?
- Do I have the unalienable right to always be treated with respect by my providers?

Now it's time to look beyond the health care system's ability to meet your individual needs and add a voice to the choir calling for transfornational change that will benefit all. Here are a few suggestions to get you started:

1. Look for opportunities to join groups that are politically active and focused on health care change. Depending on the specificity of your interest, you may elect to get involved with a national group or one that is more local.
2. Band together with like-minded individuals to establish a group within your community that is committed to high quality, low cost, safe, and equitable health care. Perhaps you will call it "Citizens Committed to Fair and Equitable Health Care." The group will need to enlist the help of individuals who have proven track records in organizing such grassroots efforts by providing leadership in such areas as

    *   articulating the group's charter and vision;
    *   attracting like-minded individuals to participate;
    *   branding the group so that it has a clear identity in the marketplace;
    *   establishing rules of engagement so that the group consistently represents a force for positive change; and
    *   building relationships with the media, health care providers, political leaders, and other key stakeholders that can give the group the leverage it needs to effect change.

    The group will need to develop a comprehensive understanding of the local health care community and its issues. As such, it will need to conduct research that provides data driven support for those issues it wishes to champion. It will need to invite the provider community to join it in dialogue. The group's objective is not chastisement but change.
3. Share your stories about encounters with the health care community—whether positive or negative. Try to conclude such stories with "lessons learned"—what you hope to accomplish by sharing your personal story with others, including:

    *   *Your provider.* Caregivers deserve an opportunity to respond to your concerns as well as be graced by your positive comments. You will learn a great deal by the way in which

providers address your issues. If you have a major concern, address it to the CEO of the hospital. If you feel the response is inadequate, consider sending all the correspondence to the chairman of the board. The chairman's fiduciary responsibility is to ensure that the hospital is serving the needs of its patients while honoring its mission.

- *Your employer.* Chances are that the company is footing most of the bill, and HR should have a strong interest in whether or not you are satisfied with the care you are receiving. You might also ask to share your story with the insurance broker or consultant that assists your company with health benefits.
- *The media.* Identify the medical writers or broadcast journalists in your market who may have an interest in your story. Journalists are often hungry for personal vignettes that provide a human touch to otherwise objective stories about health care's dysfunction.
- *Your representatives.* Tell your story to the key staff responsible for health care issues in your congressional representatives' or Senators' offices.
- *The online community.* Post your story on websites that solicit consumer feedback on experience with various providers—including Angie's List, where you can post your experience with a provider on their website, and Healthgrades.com.
- *Me.* Please consider sharing your stories with me via e-mail, and let me know if I may share them with others through publication or other means.

4. Examine the effectiveness of your state medical board to determine whether they are adequately safeguarding the public's health. If not, consider advocating with legislators to make the medical boards more effective. "Action must then be taken," insists Sidney Wolfe, MD, "legislatively and through pressure on the medical boards themselves, to increase the amount of discipline and, thus, the amount of patient protection. Without adequate legislative oversight, many medical boards will continue to perform poorly"[1]

Your participation in such "right" action, if done with an unerring intention of fulminating positive change, should prove immensely satisfying to you. Maintain your resolve, recruit others, and you will have made a difference. And if you suffer moments of doubt about assailing the medical community for its failures, remember what one of its most luminary members advised: said former *JAMA* editor George Lundberg, MD, "if some day physicians and their organizations do become primarily self-interest groups, society—which has given them the privilege of being called professionals—will rise up and take that privilege away."[2]

NOTES

MYTH I
"THE UNITED STATES BOASTS THE BEST HEALTH CARE IN THE WORLD"

1. Lawrence K. Altman, "Big Doses of Chemotherapy Drug Killed Patient, Hurt 2nd," *New York Times*, March 24, 1995, A18, http://www.nytimes.com/1995/03/24/us/big-doses-of-chemotherapy-drug-killed-patient-hurt-2d.html.

2. Ibid.

3. Ibid.

4. Christine Gorman, "The Disturbing Case of the Cure That Killed the Patient," *Time*, April 3, 1995, http://content.time.com/time/magazine/article/0,9171,982768,00.html.

5. Elizabeth Docteur and Robert A. Berenson, *How Does the Quality of U.S. Health Care Compare Internationally? Timely Analysis of Immediate Health Policy Issues* (Robert Wood Johnson Foundation, August 2009), http://www.urban.org/uploadedpdf/411947_ushealthcare_quality.pdf.

6. Docteur and Berenson, *How Does the Quality*.

7. Karen Davis, Cathy Schoen, and Kristof Stremikis, *Mirror, Mirror on the Wall: How the Performance of the U.S. Health Care System Compares Internationally* (New York: Commonwealth Foundation, 2010), http://www.commonwealthfund.org/~/media/Files/Publications/Fund Report/2010/Jun/1400_Davis_Mirror_Mirror_on_the_wall_2010.pdf.

8. Ibid., v.

9. Ibid., v.

10. Stephen Bezruchka, "Culture and Medicine: Is Globalization Danger-ous to Our Health?," *Western Journal of Medicine* 172, no. 5 (2000): 332–34, doi:10.1377/hlthaff.2012.0357, 332.

11. Docteur and Berenson, *How Does the Quality*.

12. Ibid.

13. Centers for Disease Control and Prevention, "Fast Facts: Smoking and Tobacco Use," last modified 2013, http://www.cdc.gov/tobacco/data_statistics/fact_sheets/fast_facts/.

14. Docteur and Berenson, *How Does the Quality*.

15. Institute of Medicine of the National Academies, *U.S. Health in Inter-national Perspective: Shorter Lives, Poorer Health* (Washington, D.C.: Nation-al Academies Press, 2012), 2, http://www.nap.edu/openbook.php?record_id=13497.

16. Marian F. MacDorman, Donna L. Hoyert, and T. J. Matthews, "Recent Declines in Infant Mortality in the United States, 2005–2011," *NCHS Data Brief*, no. 120 (April 2013), http://www.cdc.gov/nchs/data/databriefs/db120.pdf.

17. Ibid.

18. Institute of Medicine of the National Academies, *U.S. Health in Inter-national Perspective*.

19. Docteur and Berenson, *How Does the Quality*.

20. Ibid.

21. George D. Lundberg, *Severed Trust* (New York: Basic Books/Perseus, 2000).

22. Ibid., 19.

23. Ibid.

24. Organisation for Development and Cooperation, "OECD Health Data 2012: How Does the United States Compare," http://www.oecd.org/unitedstates/HealthSpendingInUSA_HealthData2012.pdf.

25. Davis et al., *Mirror, Mirror*.

26. David Squires, *Multinational Comparisons of Health Systems Data, 2010* (Commonwealth Fund, 2012), http://www.commonwealthfund.org/Pub-lications/Chartbooks/2011/Jul/Multinational-Comparisons-of-Health-Systems-Data-2010.aspx.

27. Derek Thompson, "Why Is American Health Care So Ridiculously Ex-pensive?," *Atlantic*, March 27, 2013, http://www.theatlantic.com/business/archive/2013/03/why-is-american-health care-so-ridiculously-expensive/274425/.

28. Robert Wood Johnson Foundation, *Consumer Attitudes on Health Care Costs: Insights from Focus Groups in Four U.S. Cities* (January 2013), http://www.rwjf.org/content/dam/farm/reports/issue_briefs/2013/rwjf403428.

29. Ibid.

30. Ibid.

31. Anne David Lassman, Benjamin Washington, Aaron Catlin, and the National Health Expenditure Accounts Team, "Growth in US Health Spending Remained Slow in 2010: Health Share of Gross Domestic Product Was Unchanged from 2009," *Health Affairs* 31, no. 1 (January 2012): 1–13, doi:10.1377/hlthaff.2011.1135.

32. Squires, *Multinational Comparisons*.

33. Ibid.

34. Ibid.

35. International Federation of Health Plans, *International Federation of Health Plans: 2012 Comparative Price Report; Variation in Medical and Hospital Prices by Country* (2012), http://hushp.harvard.edu/sites/default/files/downloadable_files/IFHP 2012 Comparative Price Report.pdf.

36. Squires, *Multinational Comparisons*.

37. T. R. Reid, *The Healing of America* (New York: Penguin, 2010).

38. International Federation of Health Plans, *International Federation of Health Plans: 2012 Comparative Price Report*.

39. Ibid.

40. Ibid.

41. Squires, *Multinational Comparisons*.

42. Ibid.

43. Docteur and Berenson, *How Does the Quality*.

44. Arnold S. Relman, *A Second Opinion* (Cambridge, Mass.: Public Affairs/Perseus Books Group, 2007), 48.

45. Davis et al., *Mirror, Mirror*.

46. Marty Makary, *Unaccountable: What Hospitals Won't Tell You and How Transparency Can Revolutionize Health Care* (New York: Bloomsbury Press, 2012), 3.

47. Linda T. Kohn, Janet M. Corrigan, and Molla S. Donaldson, *To Err Is Human: Building a Safer Health System* (Washington, D.C.: National Academy Press, 2000), 3.

48. Ibid.

49. Ibid., 2.

50. Makary, *Unaccountable*, 3.

51. World Health Organization, "World Health Report 2000: Health Systems; Improving Performance" (Geneva: World Health Organization, 2000), 1, http://www.who.int/whr/2000/en/whr00_en.pdf?ua=1.

52. Davis et al., *Mirror, Mirror*.

53. Otis Brawley, MD, in discussion with the author, August 16, 2013.

54. Lundberg, *Severed Trust*, 54.

55. Visit the AHRQ's website at http://www.ahrq.gov/research/findings/fact-sheets/minority/disparit/.

56. Agency for Healthcare Research and Quality, "Addressing Racial and Ethnic Disparities in Health Care," last modified April 2013, http://www.ahrq.gov/research/findings/factsheets/minority/disparit/.

57. Ibid.

58. Ibid.

59. Ibid.

60. Ibid.

61. Ibid.

62. Nicole Fisher, "Closing Racial and Ethnic Disparity Gaps: Implications of the Affordable Care Act," *Forbes*, last modified May 28, 2013, http://www.forbes.com/sites/theapothecary/2013/05/28/closing-racial-and-ethnic-disparity-gaps-implications-of-the-affordable-care-act/.

63. Diana Farrell, Eric Jensen, Bob Kocher, Nick Lovegrove, Fareed Melhem, Lenny Mendonca, and Beth Parish, *Accounting for the Cost of U.S. Health Care: A New Look at Why Americans Spend More*, McKinsey Global Institute, December 2008, http://www.mckinsey.com/insights/health_systems_and_services/accounting_for_the_cost_of_us_health_care.

64. Relman, *Second Opinion*, 39.

65. Ibid., 46.

66. Christine K. Cassell, "The Patient-Physician Covenant: An Affirmation of Asklepios," *Annals of Internal Medicine* 60, no. 5 (March 15, 1996): 291–93. Available online at http://www.ncbi.nlm.nih.gov/pubmed/8998907.

67. Ibid., 1.

MYTH 2
"SHOPPING FOR HEALTH CARE IS LIKE SHOPPING FOR A CAR; YOU BASE YOUR DECISIONS ON GOOD INFORMATION"

1. PWC Health Research Institute, *Scoring Healthcare: Navigating Customer Experience Ratings*, 2013. The report can be downloaded from http://www.pwc.com/us/en/health-industries/publications/scoring-patient-healthcare-experience.jhtml.

2. Peter Ubel, "How Price Transparency Could End Up Increasing health care Costs," *Atlantic*, April 2013, http://www.theatlantic.com/health/archive/2013/04/how-price-transparency-could-end-up-increasing-health care-costs/274534/.

3. Giovanni Colella, "To Bring Healthcare Prices Down, Consumers Must Demand Price Transparency," *Forbes*, March 20, 2013, http://www.forbes.

com/sites/realspin/2013/03/20/to-bring-healthcare-prices-down-consumers-must-demand-price-transparency/.

4. Ibid.

5. Pierre L. Yong, R. S. Saunders, and LeighAnne Olsen, eds., "Transparency of Cost and Performance," in *The Healthcare Imperative: Lowering Costs and Improving Outcomes: Workshop Series Summary* (Washington, D.C.: National Academy Press, 2010), available online at http://www.ncbi.nlm.nih.gov/books/NBK53921/.

6. Olga C. Damman, Michelle Hendriks, Jany Rademakers, Diana M. J. Delnoij, and Peter P. Groenewegen, "How Do Healthcare Consumers Process and Evaluate Comparative Healthcare Information? A Qualitative Study Using Cognitive Interviews," *BMC Public Health* 9, no. 423 (2009), doi:10.1186/1471-2458-9-423.

7. PWC Health Research Institute, *Scoring Healthcare*.

8. "Your Safer-Surgery Survival Guide: Our Ratings of 2,463 U.S. Hospitals Can Help You Find the Right One," *Consumer Reports*, July 2013, http://www.consumerreports.org/cro/magazine/2013/09/safe-surgery-survival-guide/index.htm.

9. *Consumer Reports'* hospital-ratings finder is available online at http://www.consumerreports.org/health/doctors-hospitals/hospital-ratings.htm.

10. S. R. Collins, Ruth Robertson, Tracy Garber, and Michelle M. Doty, "Insuring the Future: Current Trends in Health Coverage and the Effects of Implementing the Affordable Care Act," Commonwealth Fund, last modified April 2013, http://www.commonwealthfund.org/~/media/Files/Publications/Fund Report/2013/Apr/1681_Collins_insuring_future_biennial_survey_2012_FINAL.pdf.

11. Otis Brawley, MD, in discussion with the author, August 16, 2013.

12. Ibid.

13. Roseanna Sommers, Susan Dorr Goold, Elizabeth A. McGlynn, Steven D. Pearson, and Marion Danis, "Focus Groups Highlight That Many Patients Object to Clinicians' Focusing on Costs," *Health Affairs* 32, no. 2 (2012): 338–46, doi:10.1377/hlthaff.2012.0686.

14. S. R. Collins and Karen Davis, "Transparency in Health Care: The Time Has Come," Commonwealth Fund, March 15, 2006, http://www.commonwealthfund.org/Publications/Testimonies/2006/Mar/Transparency-in-health care--The-Time-Has-Come.aspx.

15. Ibid.

16. Yong, Saunders, and Olsen, "Transparency of Cost."

17. Ibid.

18. Collins and Davis, "Transparency in Health Care."

19. Michael L. Millenson, *Demanding Medical Excellence* (Chicago: University of Chicago Press, 1997), 192.

20. Marty Makary, *Unaccountable: What Hospitals Won't Tell You and How Transparency Can Revolutionize Health Care* (New York: Bloomsbury Press, 2012), 37.

21. Ibid., 39.

22. Pennsylvania Health Care Cost Containment Council, "Pennsylvania Health Care Cost Containment Council," last modified 2013, http://www.phc4.org.

23. Ibid.

24. Russ Mitchell, "29 States Get 'F' for Price Transparency Laws," *Capsules: The KHN Blog*, Kaiserhealthnews.org, March 18, 2013, http://capsules.kaiserhealthnews.org/?p=17815.

25. Catalyst for Payment Reform and Health Care Incentives Improvement Institute, *Report Card on State Price Transparency Laws*, Health Care Incentives, March 18, 2013, http://www.hci3.org/sites/default/files/files/Report_PriceTransLaws_114.pdf.

26. Uwe E. Reinhardt, "U.S. Health Care Prices Are the Elephant in the Room," *Economix*, March 29, 2013, http://economix.blogs.nytimes.com/2013/03/29/u-s-health care-prices-are-the-elephant-in-the-room/.

27. Luz Gibbons, José M. Belizán, Jeremy A. Lauer, Ana P. Betrán, Mario Merialdi, and Fernando Althabe, "The Global Numbers and Costs of Additionally Needed and Unnecessary Caesarean Sections Performed per Year: Overuse as a Barrier to Universal Coverage," World Health Organization, last modified 2010, http://www.who.int/healthsystems/topics/financing/healthreport/30C-sectioncosts.pdf.

28. Deborah Kotz, "Maternity Hospitals Push to Reduce C-Section Rate and Medical Interventions," Boston.com, October 7, 2012, http://www.boston.com/lifestyle/health/2012/10/14/maternity-hospitals-push-reduce-section-rate-and-medical-interventions/UM95Mb3oO1lLmcT0Ql4H6H/singlepage.html.

29. Ibid.

30. Fay Menacker and Brady E. Hamilton, "Recent Trends in Cesarean Delivery in the United States," Centers for Disease Control, *NCHS Data Brief*, no. 35 (March 2010), http://www.cdc.gov/nchs/data/databriefs/db35.htm.

31. Gibbons et al., "The Global Numbers and Costs."

32. Collins and Davis, "Transparency in Health Care."

33. Alain C. Enthoven, and Laura A. Tollen, "Competition in Health Care: It Takes Systems to Pursue Quality and Efficiency," *Health Affairs* (September 7, 2005): 420–33, doi:10.1377/hlthaff.w5.420.

34. Collins and Davis, "Transparency in Health Care."

35. Ibid.

36. Robert Wood Johnson Foundation, *Lessons Learned: Consumer Beliefs and Use of Information about Health Care Cost, Resource Use, and Value,* October 2012, http://www.rwjf.org/content/dam/farm/reports/issue_briefs/2012/rwjf402126.

37. Ubel, "How Price Transparency."

38. Ibid.

39. Sommers et al., "Focus Groups Highlight."

40. Ibid.

41. These sites are accessible, respectively, at https://www.healthcare.gov/where-can-i-find-provider-information/ and http://www.medicare.gov/forms-help-and-resources/find-doctors-hospitals-and-facilities/quality-care-finder.html. They are both gateway sites for http://www.medicare.gov/hospitalcompare/search.html and http://www.medicare.gov/physiciancompare/search.html.

42. Yong, Saunders, and Olsen, "Transparency of Cost."

43. Visit Florida's site at http://www.floridahealthfinder.gov/index.html.

44. Their site is found at http://hcqcc.hcf.state.ma.us/.

45. Learn more about it at http://www.uhc.com/individuals_families/member_tools/myhealthcare_cost_estimator.htm.

46. They are found at http://www.commonwealthfund.org/, http://www.rwjf.org/, and http://kff.org/, respectively.

47. And they are found online at http://www.chcf.org/ and http://www.calendow.org/, respectively.

48. Their list is available at http://caregiver.org/caregiver/jsp/fcn_content_node.jsp?nodeid=2098.

49. See https://www.healthcarebluebook.com/.

50. "Bluebook Information," Healthcare Bluebook, accessed February 26, 2014, https://healthcarebluebook.com/page_AboutHCBBMobile.aspx.

51. Arnold S. Relman, *A Second Opinion* (Cambridge, Mass.: Public Affairs/Perseus Books Group, 2007), 22–23.

MYTH 3
"MEDICAL INTERVENTIONS ARE BASED ON SCIENTIFIC EVIDENCE OF POSITIVE OUTCOMES REGARDING BEST PRACTICES; AS A RESULT, PATIENTS RECEIVE PRECISELY THE CARE THEY NEED"

1. Letitia Stein, "Desperate Families Turn to Unproven Stem Cell Treatment," *Tampa Bay Times,* May 27, 2011, http://www.tampabay.com/news/

health/medicine/desperate-families-turn-to-unproven-stem-cell-treatment/
1172182.

2. Ibid.

3. Ibid.

4. Drew Griffin and David Fitzpatrick, "US Patients Try Stem Cell Therapies Abroad," CNN.com, June 2, 2009, http://www.cnn.com/2009/HEALTH/
06/02/stem.cell.therapy/.

5. Stein, "Desperate Families."

6. Ibid.

7. Gregg Prescott, "Holistic Cancer Research: Rife Machines," Holistic
Cancer Research.com, October 2013, http://holisticcancerresearch.com/
holistic-cancer-research-rife-machine.html.

8. John Santa, "Transparency of Cost and Performance," in *The Healthcare
Imperative: Lowering Costs and Improving Outcomes: Workshop Series Summary*, ed. Pierre L. Yong, R. S. Saunders, and LeighAnne Olsen (Washington,
D.C.: National Academy Press, 2010), available online at http://www.ncbi.nlm.
nih.gov/books/NBK53921/.

9. Carolyn Newbergh, "The Dartmouth Atlas of Health Care," in *Robert
Wood Johnson Foundation Anthology: To Improve Health and Health Care*,
ed. Stephen L. Isaacs and James R. Knickman (San Francisco: Jossey-Bass,
2006), 25–48.

10. Jack A. Ginsburg, Robert B. Doherty, J. Fred Ralston Jr., and Naomi
Senkeeto, "Achieving a High Performance Health Care System with Universal
Access: What the United States Can Learn from Other Countries," *Annals of
Internal Medicine* 148, no. 1 (2008): 55-75, doi:10.7326/0003-4819-148-1-
200801010-00196.

11. J. Michael McGinnis, LeighAnne Olsen, Katharine Bothner, Daniel
O'Neill, and Dara Aisner, *Learning What Works Best: The Nation's Need for
Evidence on Comparative Effectiveness in Health Care* (Washington, D.C.:
Institute of Medicine, 2007), 1, http://www.ncbi.nlm.nih.gov/books/
NBK64784/.

12. Ibid.

13. Otis W. Brawley, *How We Do Harm: A Doctor Breaks Ranks about
Being Sick in America* (New York: St. Martin's Press, 2011), 243.

14. Ibid., 26.

15. Gabriel I. Barbash and Sherry A. Glied, "New Technology and Health
Care Costs: The Case of Robot-Assisted Surgery," *New England Journal of
Medicine* 363 (2010): 701–4, doi:10.1056/NEJMp1006602.

16. Michelle Andrews, "Questions Arise about Robotic Surgery's Cost, Effectiveness," *Kaiser Health News*, April 23, 2013, http://www.kaiserhealthnews.

org/features/insuring-your-health/2013/042313-michelle-andrews-robotic-surgery.aspx.

17. Barbash and Glied, "New Technology and Health Care."

18. Brawley, *How We Do Harm*, 204.

19. Andrews, "Questions Arise about Robotic."

20. Marty Makary, *Unaccountable: What Hospitals Won't Tell You and How Transparency Can Revolutionize Health Care* (New York: Bloomsbury Press, 2012), 155.

21. Barbash and Glied, "New Technology and Health Care."

22. Roni Caryn Rabin, "Salesmen in the Surgical Suite," *New York Times*, March 25, 2103, http://www.nytimes.com/2013/03/26/health/salesmen-in-the-surgical-suite.html.

23. Ibid., 703.

24. Makary, *Unaccountable*, 157.

25. Ibid., 155.

26. U.S. Government Accountability Office, *Higher Use of Costly Prostate Cancer Treatment by Providers Who Self-Refer Warrants Scrutiny* (Washington, D.C.: U.S. Government Accountability Office, 20130, http://www.gao.gov/products/gao 13 525.

27. Ibid.

28. Ibid.

29. Vahakn B. Shahinian, Yong-Fang Kuo, and Scott M. Gilbert. "Reimbursement Policy and Androgen-Deprivation Therapy for Prostate Cancer." *New England Journal of Medicine* 363 (November 4, 2010), doi:10.1056/NEJMsa0910784.

30. Arnold S. Relman, *A Second Opinion* (Cambridge, Mass.: Public Affairs/Perseus Books Group, 2007), 33.

31. Yong, Saunders, and Olsen, "Transparency of Cost."

32. Makary, *Unaccountable*, 4.

33. George D. Lundberg, *Severed Trust* (New York: Basic Books/Perseus, 2000), 90.

34. Brawley, *How We Do Harm*, 35.

35. Lundberg, *Severed Trust*, 262.

36. Brawley, *How We Do Harm*, 35.

37. Makary, *Unaccountable*, 151.

38. Elizabeth Docteur and Robert A. Berenson, *How Does the Quality of U.S. Health Care Compare Internationally? Timely Analysis of Immediate Health Policy Issues* (Robert Wood Johnson Foundation, August 2009), http://www.urban.org/uploadedpdf/411947_ushealthcare_quality.pdf.

39. Ibid.

40. Ibid.

41. Gardiner Harris, "Doctor Faces Suits over Cardiac Stents," *New York Times*, December 5, 2010, http://www.nytimes.com/2010/12/06/health/06stent. html.

42. Ibid.

43. David Squires, *Multinational Comparisons of Health Systems Data, 2010*, Commonwealth Fund, 2012, http://www.commonwealthfund.org/ Publications/Chartbooks/2011/Jul/Multinational-Comparisons-of-Health- Systems-Data-2010.aspx.

44. Nortin M. Hadler, *The Last Well Person: How to Stay Well Despite the Health Care System* (Montreal: McGill Queen's University Press, 2004), 20.

45. Ibid., 24.

46. Makary, *Unaccountable*, 138.

47. Hadler, *The Last Well Person*, 110.

48. Ibid., 111.

49. Brawley, *How We Do Harm*, 40.

50. Hadler, *The Last Well Person*, 78.

51. Brawley, *How We Do Harm*, 40.

52. Hadler, *The Last Well Person*, 79.

53. "Understanding of the Efficiency and Effectiveness of the Health Care System," Dartmouth Atlas of Health Care, last modified 2013, http://www. dartmouthatlas.org/.

54. Makary, *Unaccountable*, 73.

55. Otis Brawley, MD, chief medical and scientific officer, American Cancer Society, in discussion with the author, August 16, 2013.

56. Lundberg, *Severed Trust*, 18.

57. Steven Brill, "Bitter Pill: How Outrageous Pricing and Egregious Profits Are Destroying Health Care," *Time*, March 4, 2013, 16–55, https://www. scrollkit.com/s/BaSaTCZ.

58. Jason Kane, "Health Costs: How the U.S. Compares with Other Countries," *The Rundown*, PBS NewsHour, October 22, 2012, http://www.pbs.org/ newshour/rundown/2012/10/health-costs-how-the-us-compares-with-other- countries.html.

59. Ibid.

60. Brawley, *How We Do Harm*, 25.

61. Mary F. McNaughton-Collins and Michael J. Barry, "One Man at a Time: Resolving the PSA Controversy," *New England Journal of Medicine* 365 (2011): 1951–53, doi:10.1056/NEJMp1111894.

62. Hadler, *The Last Well Person*, 95.

63. Ibid., 98.

64. Andrew Pollack, "Looser Guidelines Issued on Prostate Screening," *New York Times*, May 3, 2013, http://www.nytimes.com/2013/05/04/business/prostate-screening-guidelines-are-loosened.html.

65. Brawley, *How We Do Harm*, 25.

66. Pollack, "Looser Guidelines Issued."

67. Brian Vastag, "Doctors Groups Call for End to UnnecessaryProcedures," *The Checkup* (blog), *Washington Post*, April 4, 2012. http://www.washingtonpost.com/blogs/the-checkup/post/doctors-groups-call-for-end-to-unnecessary-procedures/2012/04/03/gIQAvrDptS_blog.html.

68. Lundberg, *Severed Trust*, 11.

MYTH 4
"WHERE ONE CHOOSES TO RECEIVE CARE WILL HAVE NO BEARING ON THEIR TREATMENT OPTIONS, OUTCOMES, OR COST"

1. John Wennberg and Alan Gittelsohn, "Small Area Variations in Health Care Delivery," *Science* 182, no. 4117 (December 1973): 1102–8, doi:10.1126/science.182.4117.1102.

2. Maggie Mahar, "Braveheart," *Dartmouth Medicine*, Winter 2007, http://dartmed.dartmouth.edu/winter07/html/braveheart.php.

3. Carolyn Newbergh, "The Dartmouth Atlas of Health Care," in *Robert Wood Johnson Foundation Anthology: To Improve Health and Health Care*, ed. Stephen L. Isaacs and James R. Knickman (San Francisco: Jossey-Bass, 2006), 25–48.

4. George Lundberg, *Severed* (New York: Basic Books/Perseus, 2000), 55.

5. John E. Wennberg, "Unwarranted Variations in Healthcare Delivery: Implications for Academic Medical Centers," *British Medical Journal* 325 (October 26, 2002): 961–64, doi:http://dx.doi.org/10.1136/bmj.325.7370.961.

6. Ibid.

7. Ibid., 1105.

8. Ibid.

9. Newbergh, "The Dartmouth Atlas of Health Care," 3.

10. W. Pete Welch, Mark E. Miller, H. Gilbert Welch, Elliott S. Fisher, and John E. Wennberg, "Geographic Variation in Expenditures for Physicians' Services in the United States," *New England Journal of Medicine* 328 (March 4, 1993): 621, doi:10.1056/NEJM199303043280906.

11. Newbergh, "The Dartmouth Atlas of Health Care," 7.

12. The Dartmouth Atlas is found online at http://www.dartmouthatlas.org.

13. Shannon Brownlee, John E. Wennberg, Michael J. Barry, Elliott S. Fisher, Julie P. W. Bynum, and David C. Goodman, *Improving Patient Decision-Making in Health Care: A 2012 Dartmouth Atlas Report Highlighting the New England Region*, ed. Kristen K. Bronner (Dartmouth Institute for Health Policy & Clinical Practice, November 29, 2012), 1, http://www.dartmouthatlas. org/downloads/reports/01_Decision_Making_New_England_Region.pdf.

14. Ibid.

15. Ibid.

16. Ibid., 13–4.

17. Ibid., 37.

18. Ibid., 44.

19. Dartmouth Institute for Health Policy and Clinical Practice, "Q & A with Dr. Jack Wennberg: What's Wrong with the U.S. health care System?," last modified March 21, 2008, http://www.dartmouthatlas.org/downloads/ press/Wennberg_interviews_DartMed.pdf.

20. Ibid.

21. Brownlee et al., *Improving Patient Decision-Making in Health Care*, 9–10.

22. Ibid., 2.

23. Dartmouth Institute for Health Policy and Clinical Practice, "Q & A with Dr. Jack Wennberg."

24. John Santa, "Transparency of Cost and Performance," in *The Healthcare Imperative: Lowering Costs and Improving Outcomes: Workshop Series Summary*, ed. Pierre L. Yong, R. S. Saunders, and Leigh Anne Olsen (Washington, D.C.: National Academy Press, 2010), available online at http://www.ncbi.nlm. nih.gov/books/NBK53921/.

25. Newbergh, "The Dartmouth Atlas of Health Care," 2.

26. Wennberg, "Unwarranted Variations in Healthcare Delivery," 964.

27. Atul Gawande, "The Cost Conundrum," *New Yorker*, June 1, 2009, 6, http://www.newyorker.com/reporting/2009/06/01/090601fa_fact_gawande.

28. Ibid.

29. Brownlee et al., *Improving Patient Decision-Making in Health Care*, 3.

30. Ibid., 1.

31. Gawande, "The Cost Conundrum," 1.

32. Ibid., 2.

33. Ibid., 5–6.

34. Ibid., 12.

35. Ibid., 13.

36. Newbergh, "The Dartmouth Atlas of Health Care," 2.

37. Gawande, "The Cost Conundrum," 14.

MYTH 5
"ALL PHYSICIANS ARE CREATED EQUAL"

1. Pam Stephan, "Herlinda Garcia Survived Stage 4 Breast Cancer Misdiagnosis," About.com, July 24, 2013, http://breastcancer.about.com/b/2013/07/24/herlinda-garcia-survived-stage-4-breast-cancer-misdiagnosis.htm.

2. "Cancer-Free Woman Undergoes 7 Months of Chemotherapy after Misdiagnosis," FoxNews.com, July 18, 2013, http://www.foxnews.com/health/2013/07/18/cancer-free-woman-undergoes-7-months-chemotherapy-after-misdiagnosis/.

3. Ibid.

4. Justin Caba, "Texas Mom's Cancer Misdiagnosis: 54-Year-Old Herlinda Garcia Suffered 7 Months of Chemo, Damages Included Depression and Anxiety," *Medical Daily*, July 17, 2013, http://www.medicaldaily.com/texas-moms-cancer-misdiagnosis-54-year-old-herlinda-garcia-suffered-7-months-chemo-damages-included.

5. Stephan, "Herlinda Garcia Survived Stage 4."

6. Ibid.

7. "Cancer-Free Woman Undergoes 7 Months."

8. Brent C. James and Elizabeth H. Hammond, "The Challenge of Variation in Medical Practice," *Archive of Pathology and Laboratory Medicine* 124, no. 7 (July 2000): 1001, http://www.ncbi.nlm.nih.gov/pubmed/10888775.

9. George D. Lundberg, *Severed Trust* (New York: Basic Books/Perseus, 2000), xii.

10. David Bornstein, "Medicine's Search for Meaning," *New York Times Opinionator*, September 18, 2013, http://opinionator.blogs.nytimes.com/2013/09/18/medicines-search-for-meaning/.

11. "Best Grad Schools," Special Issue, *U.S. News & World Report*, 2014, D-95–D-105.

12. Ibid.

13. Ibid.

14. Alpha Omega Alpha Honor Medical Society, last modified 2013, http://www.alphaomegaalpha.org/.

15. "The Official Rankings of 17 Medical Departments for Their Resident Physician," last modified 1999, http://www.residentphysician.com/.

16. Marty Makary, *Unaccountable: What Hospitals Won't Tell You and How Transparency Can Revolutionize Health Care* (New York: Bloomsbury Press, 2012), 111.

17. D. A. Davis, Paul E. Mazmanian, Michael Fordis, R. Van Harrison, Kevin E. Thorpe, and Laure Perrier, "Accuracy of Physician Self-Assessment Compared with Observed Measures of Competence: A Systematic Review,"

Journal of the American Medical Association 296, no. 9 (September 6, 2006): 1094, doi:10.1001/jama.296.9.1094.

18. Nortin M. Hadler, *The Last Well Person: How to Stay Well Despite the Health Care System* (Montreal: McGill Queen's University Press, 2004), 84.

19. Makary, *Unaccountable: What Hospitals Won't Tell You*, 52.

20. Ibid.

21. Charles Inlander, cofounder of People's Medical Society, in discussion with the author, August 13, 2013.

22. Otis W. Brawley, *How We Do Harm: A Doctor Breaks Ranks about Being Sick in America* (New York: St. Martin's Press, 2011), 62.

23. Christopher Peterson and Martin Seligman, *Character Strengths and Virtues* (Oxford: Oxford University Press, 2004), 39.

24. Ibid.

25. Ibid., 100.

26. Ibid., 103.

27. Ibid., 199.

28. Ibid., 296.

29. The VIA is available online, free of charge, at http://www. authentichappiness.sas.upenn.edu/Default.aspx.

30. James and Hammond, "The Challenge of Variation," 1001.

31. Ibid., 1001.

32. Makary, *Unaccountable: What Hospitals Won't Tell You*, 102.

33. Brawley, *How We Do Harm*, 125.

34. Makary, *Unaccountable: What Hospitals Won't Tell You*, 100.

35. Peter Elias, "Sunday Dialogue: Handling Medical Errors," *New York Times*, October 18, 2013, http://www.nytimes.com/2013/10/20/opinion/sunday/sunday-dialogue-handling-medical-errors.html.

36. Makary, *Unaccountable: What Hospitals Won't Tell You*, 103–4.

37. Sidney M. Wolfe, Cynthia Williams, and Alex Zaslow, "Public Citizen's Health Research Group Ranking of the Rate of State Medical Boards' Serious Disciplinary Actions, 2009–2011," Public Citizen, last modified May 17, 2012, http://www.citizen.org/documents/2034.pdf.

38. Ibid.

39. Makary, *Unaccountable: What Hospitals Won't Tell You*, 97.

40. Ibid., 96.

41. E. V. Boisaubin and R. E. Levine, "Identifying and Assisting the Impaired Physician," *American Journal of Medical Sciences* 322, no. 1 (July 2001): 31–6, http://www.ncbi.nlm.nih.gov/pubmed/11465244.

42. Wolfe, Williams, and Zaslow, "Public Citizen's Health Research Group."

43. Lundberg, *Severed Trust*, 10.

44. Makary, *Unaccountable: What Hospitals Won't Tell You*, 102.

45. Otis Brawley, MD, chief medical and scientific officer of the American Cancer Society, in discussion with the author, August 16, 2013.

46. Arnold Milstein and Nancy E. Adler, "Out of Sight, Out of Mind: Why Doesn't Widespread Clinical Quality Failure Command Our Attention?," *Health Affairs* 22, no. 2 (2003): 119–27, http://www.ncbi.nlm.nih.gov/pubmed/12674415.

47. Ronald M. Epstein and Edward M. Hundert, "Defining and Assessing Professional Competence," *Journal of the American Medical Association* 287, no. 2 (January 9, 2002): 226–35, doi:10.1001/jama.287.2.226.

48. Ibid., 226.

49. Ibid., 227.

50. Ibid., 228.

51. Ibid., 228.

52. Ibid., 230.

53. Ibid.

54. Elisabeth Kübler-Ross, MD, author of *On Death and Dying*, in discussion with the author, September 4, 1997, Carefree, Ariz.

55. Jack A. Ginsburg, Robert B. Doherty, J. Fred Ralston Jr., and Naomi Senkeeto, "Achieving a High Performance Health Care System with Universal Access: What the United States Can Learn from Other Countries," *Annals of Internal Medicine* 148, no. 1 (2008): 59, doi:10.7326/0003-4819-148-1-200801010-00196.

56. Ken Dychtwald and Joe Flower, *Age Wave: How the Most Important Trend of Our Time Can Change Your Future* (New York: Bantam, 1990).

57. David Squires, *Multinational Comparisons of Health Systems Data, 2010*, Commonwealth Fund, 2012, http://www.commonwealthfund.org/Publications/Chartbooks/2011/Jul/Multinational-Comparisons-of-Health-Systems-Data-2010.aspx.

58. Organisation for Economic Development and Cooperation, "OECD Health Data 2010: How Does Spain Compare," June 29, 2010.

59. Organisation for Economic Development and Cooperation, "OECD Health Data 2010: How Does Canada Compare," June 29, 2010, http://www.oecd.org/els/health-systems/Briefing-Note-CANADA-2013.pdf.

60. Organisation for Economic Development and Cooperation, "OECD Health Data 2010: How Does Sweden Compare," June 29, 2010.

61. Organisation for Economic Development and Cooperation, "OECD Health Data 2010: How Does Germany Compare," June 29, 2010.

62. Doug Henley, MD, CEO of American Academy of Family Physicians, in discussion with the author, November 7, 2013, Leawood, Kans.

63. Ibid.

64. Charles Inlander in discussion with the author, August 13, 2013.

65. Doug Henley, MD, in discussion with the author, November 7, 2013, Leawood, Kans.

66. American Academy of Family Physicians, last modified 2013, http://www.aafp.org/home.html.

67. Intermountain Health Care, last modified 2013, http://intermountainhealthcare.org/providers/specialties.html.

68. Ibid.

69. Otis Brawley, MD, in discussion with the author, August 16, 2013.

70. Ibid.

71. DocFinder is found online at http://www.docboard.org/docfinder.html.

72. Brawley, *How We Do Harm*, 52.

MYTH 6
"THERE'S NO BETTER PLACE TO BE WHEN YOU ARE ILL THAN THE HOSPITAL"

1. "Doctor Who Cut Off Wrong Leg Is Defended by Colleagues," *New York Times*, September 17, 1995, http://www.nytimes.com/1995/09/17/us/doctor-who-cut-off-wrong-leg-is-defended-by-colleagues.html.

2. Sandra G. Boodman, "The Pain of Wrong Site Surgery," *Washington Post*, June 20, 2011, http://articles.washingtonpost.com/2011-06-20/national/35235752_1_wrong-site-surgery-wrong-site-surgery-universal-protocol.

3. Walt Bogdanich, "Viewpoint," *The Leifer Report*, Spring 1992, 6–7.

4. National Association of Public Hospitals and Health Systems, "History of Public Hospitals and Health Systems," last modified 2013, http://www.naph.org/Homepage-Sections/Explore/History.aspx.

5. Arnold S. Relman, *A Second Opinion* (Cambridge, Mass.: Public Affairs/Perseus Books Group, 2007), 58.

6. Ibid., 57–58.

7. Phil Cohen, "Deming's 14 Points," HCi, http://www.hci.com.au/hcisite2/articles/deming.htm.

8. "Guru: W. Edwards Deming," *Economist*, last modified June 5, 2009. http://www.economist.com/node/13805735.

9. Donald M. Berwick, "Controlling Variation in Health Care: A Consultation from Walter Shewhart," *Medical Care* 29, no. 12 (December 1991): 1212.

10. Amir A. Ghaferi, John D. Birkmeyer, and Justin B. Dimick, "Variation in Hospital Mortality Associated with Inpatient Surgery," *New England Journal of Medicine* 361 (October 1, 2009): 1368–75, doi:10.1056/NEJM-sa0903048.

11. Ibid., 1370.

12. Chelsea Conaboy, "Report: Variations in Quality of Care a 'Hidden' Curriculum for New Doctors at Teaching Hospitals," *Boston Globe*, October 30, 2012, http://www.boston.com/whitecoatnotes/2012/10/30/report-variations-quality-care-hidden-curriculum-for-new-doctors-teaching-hospitals/CGdrLdXtCgy3qFJwhi7t9I/story.html.

13. "Mass General Hospital Ranked No. 1," Harvard Medical School, July 17, 2012, http://hms.harvard.edu/news/mass-general-hospital-ranked-no-1-7-17-12.

14. Olivia Victoria Andrzejczak, "Lawsuit: TV Producer Pumped Full of Drugs," Timesunion.com, August 9, 2009, http://www.timesunion.com/local/article/Dead-by-mistake-547833.php.

15. Olivia Victoria Andrzejczak, "60 Minutes' Ace's Death Echoes of His Own Investigations," *Houston Chronicle*, July 30, 2009, http://www.chron.com/news/article/60-Minutes-ace-s-death-echoes-his-own-1747718.php.

16. Sanjay Marwah and Sham Lal Singla, "Spirit-Induced Cautery Burns: An Unusual Iatrogenic Injury," *Internet Journal of Surgery* 22, no. 2 (2010). 1, http://ispub.com/IJS/22/2/9414.

17. Sonya P. Mehta, Sanjay M. Bhananker, Karen L. Posner, and Karen B. Domino, "Operating Room Fires: A Closed Claims Analysis," *Anesthesiology* 118, no. 5: 1133-39, doi: 10.1097/ALN.0b013e31828afa7b.

18. Mehta et al., "Operating Room Fires," 17.

19. Theodore Kim and Tammy Webber, "Third Baby Dies after Error at Indiana Hospital," *USA Today*, September 20, 2006, http://usatoday30.usatoday.com/news/nation/2006-09-20-baby-deaths_x.htm.

20. Ibid.

21. Laura A. Fahrenthold, "4-yr.-old Dies after Surgery," *New York Daily News*, March 23, 1995, http://www.nydailynews.com/archives/news/4-yr-old-dies-surgery-article-1.688316.

22. John Bonifield, "Ohio Family: Hospital 'Botched' Transplant, Threw Out Kidney," CNN, August 30, 2013, http://www.cnn.com/2013/08/30/health/transplant-kidney-thrown-away/.

23. Susan Donaldson James, "Toledo Hospital Threw Out Donor Kidney, Now Denies Negligence," ABCNews, August 29, 2013, http://abcnews.go.com/Health/toledo-hospital-threw-donor-kidney-now-denies-negligence/story?id=20110334.

24. Sara Bleich, "Medical Errors: Five Years after the IOM Report," Commonwealth Fund, last modified July 2005, http://www.commonwealthfund.org/usr_doc/830_bleich_errors.pdf.

25. Ibid., 9.

26. Kiernan Walshe and Stephen M. Shortell, "When Things Go Wrong: How Health Care Organizations Deal with Major Failures," *Health Affairs* 23, no. 3 (May 2004): 107, http://content.healthaffairs.org/content/23/3/103.full.

27. Ibid.

28. Jim Doyle, "Blunders: Botched Brain Surgery Prompts Extensive Review at SSM Health Care," *St. Louis Post Dispatch*, May 5, 2013, http://www.stltoday.com/business/local/botched-brain-surgery-prompts-extensive-review-at-ssm-health care/article_df1f66b8-ba03-5ba1-8e93-ce0cc771f0a5.html.

29. Bleich, "Medical Errors," 9.

30. Denise Grady, "Hospitals Profit from Surgical Errors, Study Finds," *New York Times*, April 17, 2013, http://www.nytimes.com/2013/04/17/health/hospitals-profit-from-surgical-errors-study-finds.html.

31. Sule Calikoglu, Robert Murray, and Dianne Feeney, "Hospital Pay-for-Performance Programs in Maryland Produced Strong Results, Including Reduced Hospital-Acquired Conditions," *Health Affairs* 31, no. 12 (December 2012): 2653, doi:10.1377/hlthaff.2012.0357.

32. Charles Babcock, "Data on Hospital Errors to Be Deleted," *Boston Globe*, May 3, 2013, http://www.bostonglobe.com/news/nation/2013/05/02/delete-data-life-threatening-hospital-mistakes-from-website/LkVNaa9CKBlQmMIwODdvWI/story.html.

33. Steven Brill, "Bitter Pill: How Outrageous Pricing and Egregious Profits Are Destroying Health Care," *Time*, March 4, 2013: 3, https://www.scrollkit.com/s/BaSaTCZ.

34. Anne Martin, David Lassman, Benjamin Washington, Aaron Catlin, and the National Health Expenditure Accounts Team, "Growth in US Health Spending Remained Slow in 2010; Health Share of Gross Domestic Product Was Unchanged from 2009," *Health Affairs* 31, no. 1 (January 2012), doi:10.1377/hlthaff.2011.1135.

35. Ibid.

36. Nina Bernstein, "How to Charge $546 for Six Liters of Saltwater," *New York Times*, August 25, 2013, http://www.nytimes.com/2013/08/27/health/exploring-salines-secret-costs.html.

37. Rich Daly, "CMS Data Show Wide Variation in Hospital Billing," *Modern Healthcare*, last modified May 8, 2013, 213, http://www.modernhealthcare.com/article/20130508/NEWS/305089960#.

38. Christopher P. Tompkins, Stuart H. Altman, and Efrat Eilat, "The Precarious Pricing System for Hospital Services," *Health Affairs* 25, no. 1 (January–February 2006): 48, doi:10.1377/hlthaff.25.1.45.

39. Brill, "Bitter Pill," 37–38.

40. Ibid., 26.

41. T. R. Reid, *The Healing of America* (New York: Penguin, 2010), 91.

42. Ibid., 92.

43. Ibid., 84.

44. Brill, "Bitter Pill," 22.

45. Ibid., 29.

46. Tompkins, Altman, and Eilat, "The Precarious Pricing System," 54.

47. Brill, "Bitter Pill," 55.

48. Robert Wood Johnson Foundation, *Lessons Learned: Consumer Beliefs and Use of Information about Health Care Cost, Resource Use, and Value*, October 2012, http://www.rwjf.org/content/dam/farm/reports/issue_briefs/2012/rwjf402126.

49. Walshe and Shortell, "When Things Go Wrong," 110.

50. Ibid., 107.

51. Julic Creswell and Reed Abelson, "New Laws and Rising Costs Create a Surge in Supersizing Hospitals," *New York Times*, August 12, 2013, http://www.nytimes.com/2013/08/13/business/bigger-hospitals-may-lead-to-bigger-bills-for-patients.html.

52. "Saint Luke's Health System CEO Hastings Will Retire," *Kansas City Business Journal*, January 12, 2011, http://www.bizjournals.com/kansascity/news/2011/01/12/saint-lukes-health-system-cco.html.

53. Marty Makary, *Unaccountable: What Hospitals Won't Tell You and How Transparency Can Revolutionize Health Care* (New York: Bloomsbury Press, 2012), 129.

54. Brill, "Bitter Pill," 40.

55. Makary, *Unaccountable: What Hospitals Won't Tell You*, 147.

56. Healthcare Bluebook is found online at http://www.healthcarebluebook.com.

57. Jeff Rice, MD, president of Healthcare Bluebook, in discussion with the author, August 16, 2013.

58. Ibid.

59. Ibid.

60. Ibid.

MYTH 7
"THE PRESCRIPTION I WAS GIVEN IS SAFE, PROVEN, AND EFFECTIVE"

1. Jonathan Mahler, "The Antidepressant Dilemma," *New York Times*, November 21, 2004, http://www.nytimes.com/2004/11/21/magazine/21TEENS.html?pagewanted=all&position=&_r=0.

2. Ibid.

3. Ibid.

4. Ibid.

5. Ibid.

6. Ben Goldacre, "Trial sans Error: How Pharma-Funded Research Cherry-Picks Positive Results [Excerpt]," *Scientific American*, February 13, 2013, 2, http://www.scientificamerican.com/article.cfm?id=trial-sans-error-how-pharma-funded-research-cherry-picks-positive-results.

7. Ibid.

8. Rob Garver and Charles Seife, "FDA Lets Drugs Approved on Fraudulent Research Stay on the Market," ProPublica, last modified April 15, 2013, http://www.propublica.org/article/fda-let-drugs-approved-on-fraudulent-research-stay-on-the-market.

9. Ibid.

10. Ibid.

11. Ibid.

12. Rob Garver and Charles Seife, "Double Dose: In Second Case of Flawed Drug Research, FDA Response Was Slow and Secretive," ProPublica, last modified April 17, 2013, http://www.propublica.org/article/double-dose-in-second-case-of-flawed-drug-research-fda-response-was-slow.

13. Ibid.

14. Ibid., 2.

15. Ibid.

16. Goldacre, "Trial sans Error," 2.

17. Ibid., 8.

18. Ibid., 8.

19. Ibid., 3.

20. Ibid.

21. Ibid.

22. Nortin M. Hadler, *The Last Well Person: How to Stay Well Despite the Health Care System* (Montreal: McGill Queen's University Press, 2004), 35.

23. Goldacre, "Trial sans Error," 1.

24. Ibid., 2.

25. Ibid., 5.

26. Anthony L. Zietman, "Falsification, Fabrication, and Plagiarism: The Unholy Trinity of Scientific Writing," *International Journal of Radiation Oncology* 87, no. 2 (October 1, 2013): 225, http://www.elsevier.com/connect/falsification-fabrication-and-plagiarism-the-unholy-trinity-of-scientific-writing.

27. Marcia Angell, "Excess in the Pharmaceutical Industry," *Canadian Medical Association Journal* 171, no. 12 (December 7, 2004), doi:10.1503/cmaj.1041594.

28. Rick Newman, "Why Health Insurers Make Lousy Villains," *MONEY*, *USNews.com*, August 25, 2009, http://money.usnews.com/money/blogs/flowchart/2009/08/25/why-health-insurers-make-lousy-villains.

29. Ibid.

30. Ezra Klein, "Health-Insurance Industry: Still Not That Profitable," *Washington Post*, February 24, 2011, http://voices.washingtonpost.com/ezra-klein/2011/02/health-insurance_industry_stil.html.

31. Vivian Hunt, Nigel Manson, and Paul Morgan, "A Wake-Up Call for Big Pharma," McKinsey & Company, last modified December 2011, http://www.mckinsey.com/insights/health_systems/a_wake-up_call_for_big_pharma.

32. Katie Thomas, "U.S. Drug Costs Dropped in 2012, but Rises Loom," *New York Times*, March 18, 2013, http://www.nytimes.com/2013/03/19/business/use-of-generics-produces-an-unusual-drop-in-drug-spending.html.

33. *Association for Molecular Pathology et al. v. Myriad Genetics, Inc. et al.*, 569 U.S. 12-398 (2013), http://www.law.cornell.edu/supremecourt/text/12-398-writing-12-398_SYLLABUS.

34. Rachel Kornfield, Julie Donohue, Ernst. R. Berndt, and G. Caleb Alexander, "Promotion of Prescription Drugs to Consumer and Providers, 2001–2010," *PLOS ONE* 8, no. 3 (March 4, 2013): 3, http://www.plosone.org/article/info%3Adoi%2F10.1371%2Fjournal.pone.0055504.

35. D. W. McFadden, E. Calvario, and C. Graves, "The Devil Is in the Details: The Pharmaceutical Industry's Use of Gifts to Physicians as Marketing Strategy," *Journal of Surgical Research* 140, no. 1 (June 1, 2007): 1, http://www.ncbi.nlm.nih.gov/pubmed/17481979.

36. Kornfield, Donohue, Berndt, and Alexander, "Promotion of Prescription Drugs," 1.

37. Ibid.

38. Ibid., 2.

39. Dana Katz, Arthur L. Caplan, and Jon F. Merz, "All Gifts Large and Small," *American Journal of Bioethics* 3, no. 3 (Summer 2003): 11, available online at http://repository.upenn.edu/cgi/viewcontent.cgi?article=1050&context=bioethics_papers.

40. Roni Caryn Rabin, "Doctors' Lucrative Industry Ties," *Well* (blog), *New York Times*, May 13, 2013, http://well.blogs.nytimes.com/2013/05/13/doctors-lucrative-industry-ties/.

41. Emily Ramshaw and Ryan Murphy, "Payments to Doctors by Pharmaceutical Companies Raise Conflicts of Interest," *New York Times*, November 24, 2011, http://www.nytimes.com/2011/11/25/us/payments-to-doctors-by-pharmaceutical-companies-raise-issues-of-conflicts.html.

42. Rabin, "Doctors' Lucrative Industry Ties."

43. Pauline W. Chen, "For Med Students, Love from the Drug Rep," *Well*, October 3, 2013, http://well.blogs.nytimes.com/2013/10/03/for-med-students-love-from-the-drug-rep/.

44. Katz, Caplan, and Merz, "All Gifts Large and Small," 7.

45. Ashley Wazana, "Physicians and the Pharmaceutical Industry: Is a Gift Ever Just a Gift?," *Journal of the American Medical Association* 283, no. 3 (January 19, 2000): 373, doi:10.1001/jama.283.3.373.

46. Ibid.

47. Robert Steinbrook, "Disclosure of Industry Payments to Physicians," *New England Journal of Medicine* 359, no. 6 (August 7, 2008): 559, available online at http://depts.washington.edu/hmcderma/Steinbrook_NEJM-08.pdf.

48. Ramshaw and Murphy, "Payments to Doctors by Pharmaceutical Companies."

49. Katz, Caplan, and Merz, "All Gifts Large and Small."

50. D. Korenstein, A. S. Keyhani, and S. Ross, "Physician Attitudes toward Industry: A View across the Specialties," *Archives of Surgery* 145, no. 6 (June 2010): 571, doi:10.1001/archsurg.2010.75.

51. Ibid., 572.

52. Ibid., 571.

53. Rabin, "Doctors' Lucrative Industry Ties."

54. Jennifer Neuman, Deborah Korenstein, Joseph S. Ross, and Salomeh Keyhani, "Prevalence of Financial Conflicts of Interest among Panel Members Producing Clinical Practice Guidelines in Canada and the United States: Cross Sectional Study," *British Medical Journal* 343 (2011): d5621 doi: 10.1136/bmj.d5621 (all quotations from the first page), http://dx.doi.org/10.1136/bmj.d5621.

55. Ibid.

56. Donna U. Vogt, *CRS Report for Congress: Direct to Consumer Advertising of Prescription Drugs* (Washington, D.C.: Library of Congress, March 25, 2005), available online at http://www.law.umaryland.edu/marshall/crsreports/crsdocuments/RL3285303252005.pdf.

57. Kornfield, Donohue, Berndt, and Alexander, "Promotion of Prescription Drugs," 2.

58. Barbara Mintzes, Morris L. Barer, Richard L. Kravitz, Ken Bassett, Joel Lexchin, Arminée Kazanjian, Robert G. Evans, Richard Pan, and Stephen A. Marion, "How Does Direct-to-Consumer Advertising (DTCA) Affect Prescribing? A Survey in Primary Care Environments with and without Legal DTCA," *Canadian Medical Association Journal* 169, no. 5 (September 2, 2003): 408, http://www.ncbi.nlm.nih.gov/pmc/articles/PMC183290/.

59. Vogt, *CRS Report for Congress*, 3.

60. Ibid.

61. Paul H. Keckley, *Deloitte 2012 Survey of U.S. Health Care Consumers: The Performance of the Health Care System and Health Care Reform*, Deloitte, 2012, http://www.deloitte.com/assets/dcom-unitedstates/local assets/ documents/health reform issues briefs/us_chs_issuebrief_2012consumersurvey_061212.pdf.

62. Elisabeth Rosenthal, "A Push to Sell Testosterone Gels Troubles Doctors," *New York Times*, October 15, 2013, http://www.nytimes.com/2013/10/16/ us/a-push-to-sell-testosterone-gels-troubles-doctors.html.

63. Ibid.

64. Otis W. Brawley, *How We Do Harm: A Doctor Breaks Ranks about Being Sick in America* (New York: St. Martin's Press, 2011), 72.

65. Ibid., 73.

66. Ibid., 85.

67. Ibid., 73.

68. Ibid., 97.

69. Andrew Pollack, "Doctors Denounce Cancer Drug Prices of $100,000 a Year," *New York Times*, April 25, 2013, http://www.nytimes.com/2013/04/26/ business/cancer-physicians-attack-high-drug-costs.html.

70. Ibid.

71. YahooNews, "The Sky-High Price of Chemotherapy: Why Do Cancer Drugs Cost So Much?," last modified May 9, 2013, http://news.yahoo.com/sky-high-price-chemotherapy-why-cancer-drugs-cost-223821525.html.

72. Pollack, "Doctors Denounce Cancer Drug Prices."

73. Public Citizen, "The Other Drug War: Big Pharma's 625 Washington Lobbyists," last modified July 23, 2001, http://www.citizen.org/documents/ pharmadrugwar.PDF.

74. Ibid.

75. Open Secrets.org, Center for Responsive Politics, "Lobbying: Pharmaceuticals/Health Products," last modified 2013, http://www.opensecrets.org/ lobby/indusclient.php?id=H04.

76. Ibid.

77. Ibid.

78. Ibid.

79. "Another Alleged Drug Kickback Scheme," *New York Times*, April 27, 2013, http://www.nytimes.com/2013/04/28/opinion/sunday/another-alleged-drug-kickback-scheme.html.

80. Ibid.

81. Ibid.

82. J. T. LaFleur, Weber, C. Ornstein, and J. Larson, "How We Analyzed Medicare's Drug Data," ProPublica, May 11, 2013, http://www.propublica.org/ article/how-we-analyzed-medicares-drug-data-long-methodology.

83. Tracy Weber and C. Ornstein, "Why You Should Care about the Drugs Your Doctor Prescribes," ProPublica, July 15, 2013, http://www.propublica.org/article/why-you-should-care-about-the-drugs-your-doctor-prescribes.

84. Ibid.

85. Elizabeth J. Cappiello, "Physician Payments Sunshine Act," *Health Law Alert News Letter* 2 (2010), Ober Kaler Attorneys at Law, last modified 2010, http://www.ober.com/publications/1101-physician-payment-sunshine-act.

86. Visit http://www.nlm.nih.gov/medlineplus/druginformation.html.

87. Visit http://www.drugs.com.

88. Visit http://www.webmd.com/.

89. Visit http://www.fda.gov/Drugs/default.htm.

90. Visit http://www.mayoclinic.com/health/drug-information/DrugHerbIndex.

91. Visit http://www.cvs.com/drug/information.jsp.

92. Visit http://naturaldatabaseconsumer.therapeuticresearch.com/home.aspx.

93. Visit http://www.fda.gov/healthfraud.

94. "Dangerous Supplements: What You Don't Know about These 12 Supplements Could Hurt You," *Consumer Reports*, last modified May 2012, http://www.consumerreports.org/cro/2012/05/dangerous-supplements/.

MYTH 8
"I'M JUST THE PATIENT; I'M NOT PART OF THE PROBLEM"

1. Centers for Disease Control and Prevention, "Chronic Diseases and Health Promotion," last modified August 13, 2012, http://www.cdc.gov/chronicdisease/overview/index.htm.

2. James F. Fries, "Aging, Natural Death, and the Compression of Morbidity," *New England Journal of Medicine* 303 (July 17, 1980): 132, doi:10.1056/NEJM198007173030304.

3. Ibid., 248.

4. Ibid.

5. Centers for Disease Control and Prevention, "Chronic Diseases and Health Promotion."

6. Institute of Medicine of the National Academies, *U.S. Health in International Perspective: Shorter Lives, Poorer Health* (Washington, D.C.: National Academies Press, 2012), http://www.nap.edu/openbook.php?record_id=13497.

7. John L. Ratey with Eric Hagerman, *Spark: The Revolutionary New Science of Exercise and the Brain* (New York: Little, Brown and Company, 2008).

8. American Psychological Association, "Ray's Race: Running Psychologists Presents the 34th Annual Ray's Race 5K Run and Walk," last modified May 2012, www.apa.org/about/division/officers/dialogue/2012/05/rays-race.aspx.

9. Janet S. Hildebrand, Susan M. Gapstur, Peter T. Campbell, Mia M. Gaudet, and Alpa V. Patel, "Recreational Physical Activity and Leisure-Time Sitting in Relation to Postmenopausal Breast Cancer Risk," *Cancer Epidemiology, Biomarkers & Prevention*, October 22, 2013, doi: 10.1158/1055-9965.EPI-13-0407.

10. Nathan Bomey, "University of Michigan Wellness Pioneer Dee Edington Launches Startup," *Ann Arbor News*, October 23, 2012, http://www.annarbor.com/business-review/university-of-michigan-wellness-pioneer-dee-edington-launches-startup/.

11. Section 4103 of the ACA, as paraphrased by Centers for Disease Control and Prevention, "A Framework for Patient-Centered Health Risk Assessments," last modified December 12, 2011, http://www.cdc.gov/policy/opth/hra/.

MYTH 9
"MY INSURANCE COMPANY'S FIRST CONCERN IS MY HEALTH"

1. Matt Gertz, "Nets Ignore Testimony of Cancer Patient Denied Coverage by Insurer," Media Matters, June 22, 2009, http://mediamatters.org/research/2009/06/22/nets-ignore-testimony-of-cancer-patient-denied/151406.

2. "Cancer Patient Tells of Rips in Health Insurance Safety Net," CNN.com, June 16, 2009, http://www.cnn.com/2009/POLITICS/06/16/health.care.hearing/.

3. Ibid.

4. Ibid.

5. Ibid.

6. Department for Professional Employees AFL-CIO, "2012 Fact Sheet: The U.S. Health Care System: An International Perspective," last modified April 2012, http://dpeaflcio.org/wp-content/uploads/US-health care-in-Intl-Perspective-2012.pdf.

7. Kaiser Family Foundation, "Employer Health Benefits 2010 Summary of Findings," September 2010, 1.

8. Ibid.

9. J. Michael McGinnis, LeighAnne Olsen, Katharine Bothner, Daniel O'Neill, and Dara Aisner, *Learning What Works Best: The Nation's Need for Evidence on Comparative Effectiveness in Health Care* (Washington, D.C.: Institute of Medicine, 2007), 2, http://www.ncbi.nlm.nih.gov/books/NBK64784/.

10. Kaiser Family Foundation and Health Research and Educational Trust, "Employer Health Benefits: 2012 Annual Survey," last modified September 11, 2012, 1, http://kaiserfamilyfoundation.files.wordpress.com/2013/03/8345-employer-health-benefits-annual-survey-full-report-0912.pdf.

11. Cathy Schoen, Jacob Lippa, Sara Collins, and David Radley, "State Trends in Premiums and Deductibles, 2003–2011: Eroding Protection and Rising Costs Underscore Need for Action," Commonwealth Fund, last modified December 2012, http://www.commonwealthfund.org/Publications/Issue-Briefs/2012/Dec/State-Trends-in-Premiums-and-Deductibles.aspx.

12. Health Care Incentives Improvement Institute (HCI3), "Affordability of Health Care: Metrics for Tranformation," last modified 2012, http://www.hci3.org/content/affordability-health care-metrics-transformation.

13. Schoen et al., "State Trends in Premiums," 2.

14. Andrew Pollack, "Health Care Costs Climb Moderately, Survey Says," *New York Times*, August 20, 2013, http://www.nytimes.com/2013/08/21/business/survey-finds-modest-rise-in-health-insurance-premiums.html.

15. Jack A. Ginsburg, Robert B. Doherty, J. Fred Ralston Jr., and Naomi Senkeeto, "Achieving a High Performance Health Care System with Universal Access: What the United States Can Learn from Other Countries," *Annals of Internal Medicine* 148, no. 1 (2008): 55–75, doi:10.7326/0003-4819-148-1-200801010-00196.

16. Schoen et al., "State Trends in Premiums," 3.

17. Kaiser Family Foundation and Health Research and Educational Trust, "Employer Health Benefits: 2012," 3.

18. Ibid., 2.

19. Kaiser Family Foundation and Health Research and Educational Trust, "Employer Health Benefits: 2012," 5.

20. Schoen et al., "State Trends in Premiums," 1.

21. Ibid., 2.

22. Kaiser Family Foundation and Health Research and Educational Trust, "Employer Health Benefits: 2012," 1.

23. Hubert Janicki, "Employment-Based Health Insurance: 2010," United States Census Bureau/U.S. Department of Commerce, last modified February 2013, 2, http://www.census.gov/prod/2013pubs/p70-134.pdf.

24. Ibid., 8.

25. Schoen et al., "State Trends in Premiums," 3.

26. Centers for Disease Control and Prevention, "FASTSTATS: Health Insurance Coverage," last modified August 20, 2012, 1, http://www.cdc.gov/nchs/fastats/hinsure.htm.

27. Ibid.

28. Kaiser Family Foundation, "The Uninsured and the Difference Health Insurance Makes," September 1, 2012, http://kff.org/uninsured/fact-sheet/the-uninsured-and-the-difference-health-insurance/.

29. Centers for Disease Control and Prevention, "FASTSTATS: Health Insurance Coverage," 4, http://www.cdc.gov/nchs/data/nhis/earlyrelease/insur201206.pdf.

30. Elizabeth Docteur and Robert A. Berenson, *How Does the Quality of U.S. Health Care Compare Internationally? Timely Analysis of Immediate Health Policy Issues* (Robert Wood Johnson Foundation, August 2009), http://www.urban.org/uploadedpdf/411947_ushealthcare_quality.pdf.

31. Robert Wood Johnson Foundation, *Consumer Attitudes on Health Care Costs: Insights from Focus Groups in Four U.S. Cities*, January 2013, http://www.rwjf.org/content/dam/farm/reports/issue_briefs/2013/rwjf403428.

32. Ibid.

33. Ibid.

34. S. R. Collins, Ruth Robertson, Tracy Garber, and Michelle M. Doty, "Insuring the Future: Current Trends in Health Coverage and the Effects of Implementing the Affordable Care Act," Commonwealth Fund, last modified April 2013, http://www.commonwealthfund.org/~/media/Files/Publications/FundReport/2013/Apr/1681 Collins_insuring_future_biennial_survey_2012_FINAL.pdf, xii.

35. Schoen et al., "State Trends in Premiums," 2.

36. "Update on Health Care Reform," *Consumer Reports*, last modified March 2013, http://www.consumerreports.org/cro/2012/06/update-on-healthcare-reform/index.htm.

37. Connie Cass and Ricardo Alonso-Zaldivar, "What Now? Q & A about Latest Snag in Health Care Law," *Associated Press*, July 4, 2013, http://bigstory.ap.org/article/what-now-qa-about-latest-snag-health care-law.

38. Robert Pear, "A Limit on Consumer Costs Is Delayed in Health Care Law," *New York Times*, August 12, 2013, http://www.nytimes.com/2013/08/13/us/a-limit-on-consumer-costs-is-delayed-in-health care-law.html.

39. Russ Douthat, "Obamacare, Failing Ahead of Schedule," *New York Times*, October 19, 2013, http://www.nytimes.com/2013/10/20/opinion/sunday/douthat-obamacare-failing-ahead-of-schedule.html.

40. "Update on Health Care Reform," *Consumer Reports*.

41. Schoen et al., "State Trends in Premiums," 9.

42. Visit https://www.healthcare.gov/what-are-my-preventive-care-benefits/.

43. Schoen et al., "State Trends in Premiums," 3.

44. G. Collins, "Frankenstein Goes to Congress," *New York Times*, October 4, 2013, http://www.nytimes.com/2013/10/05/opinion/collins-frankenstein-goes-to-congress.html.

45. S. R. Collins et al., "Insuring the Future."

46. Sarah Frier, "Insurers Profit from Health Law They Fought Against," Bloomberg, last modified January 5, 2012, http://www.bloomberg.com/news/2012-01-05/health-insurer-profit-rises-as-obama-s-health-law-supplies-revenue-boost.html.

47. Ibid.

48. Health Care for America Now, "Health Insurance Industry," October 4, 2013, http://healthcareforamericanow.org/ourissues/health-insurance-industry/.

49. "CEO Compensation, 2012," *Forbes*, December 2012, http://www.forbes.com/lists.

50. Jay Hancock, "Health Insurance Actuaries in the Hot Seat on 'Rate Shock," Kaiser Health News, April 18, 2013, http://www.kaiserhealthnews.org/stories/2013/april/18/actuaries-ties-to-insurance-rate-shock.aspx.

51. Ibid.

52. Ibid.

53. "FDA Approval for Bevacizumab," National Cancer Institute, October 2013, http://www.cancer.gov/cancertopics/druginfo/fda-bevacizumab.

54. Families USA, "Resources for Consumers," last modified July 2011, http://www.familiesusa.org/resources/resources-for-consumers/.

55. Medicare.gov, "How Do I File an Appeal?," visited July 5, 2013, http://www.medicare.gov/claims-and-appeals/file-an-appeal/appeals.html.

56. Visit http://www.nolo.com/legal-encyclopedia/how-appeal-denial-medicaid-non-eligibility.html.

MYTH 10
"WHEN ALL ELSE FAILS, AT LEAST THE SYSTEM WILL ALLOW ME TO DIE WITH DIGNITY"

1. George D. Lundberg, *Severed Trust* (New York: Basic Books/Perseus, 2000), 221.

2. Otis W. Brawley, *How We Do Harm: A Doctor Breaks Ranks about Being Sick in America* (New York: St. Martin's Press, 2011), 122.

3. Lundberg, *Severed Trust*, 231.

4. Elisabeth Kübler-Ross, *On Death and Dying* (New York: Macmillan Publishing, 1969), 7.

5. Robert Frost, "The Road Not Taken," available online at http://www.poetryfoundation.org/poem/173536.

6. A. Smith, K. E. McCarthy, E. Weber, I. S. Cenzer, J. Boscardin, J. Fisher, and K. Covinsky, "Half of Older Americans Seen in Emergency Department in Last Month of Life: Most Admitted to Hospital, and Many Die There," *Health Affairs* 31, no. 7 (May 31, 2013): 1297, doi:10.1377/hlthaff.2011.0922.

7. Kübler-Ross, *On Death and Dying*, 8.

8. Ira Byock, *Dying Well* (New York: Riverhead, 1997), 27.

9. Smith et al., "Half of Older Americans," 1280.

10. Lundberg, *Severed Trust*, 238.

11. Ibid., 232.

12. Ibid., 12.

13. Kübler-Ross, *On Death and Dying*, 9.

14. Lundberg, *Severed Trust*, 2.

15. Kübler-Ross, *On Death and Dying*, 6.

16. Byock, *Dying Well*, 23.

17. Ibid., 25–26.

18. Kübler-Ross, *On Death and Dying*, 11.

19. Lundberg, *Severed Trust*, 221.

20. Elisabeth Kübler-Ross, MD, author of *On Death and Dying*, in discussion with the author, September 4, 1997, Carefree, Ariz.

21. Ibid.

22. Lundberg, *Severed Trust*, 12.

23. Brawley, *How We Do Harm*, 122.

24. Carolyn Newbergh, "The Dartmouth Atlas of Health Care," in *Robert Wood Johnson Foundation Anthology: To Improve Health and Health Care*, ed. Stephen L. Isaacs and James R. Knickman (San Francisco: Jossey-Bass, 2006), 9.

25. Dartmouth Atlas of Health Care, "Care of Chronic Illness in the Last Two Years of Life," last modified 2013, http://www.dartmouthatlas.org/data/topic/topic.aspx?cat=1.

26. Marilyn J. Field and Christine K. Cassell, *Approaching Death: Improving Care at the End of Life* (Washington, D.C.: National Academy Press, 1997), 2.

27. Ira Byock, *Dying Well* (New York: Riverhead, 1997), 60.

28. Smith et al., "Half of Older Americans," 1282.

29. Ann Carrns, "Deciding When to Enter a Palliative Care Unit," *New York Times*, September 4, 2013, http://www.nytimes.com/2013/09/04/your-money/deciding-when-to-enter-a-palliative-care-unit.html.

30. Elisabeth Kübler-Ross, MD, in discussion with the author, September 4, 1997, Carefree, Ariz.

31. Byock, *Dying Well*, 57.

32. This document may be found in its entirety at http://uofmhealthsystem. org/documents/adult/AdvanceDirectiveBooklet.pdf.

33. Kate O'Malley and Nancy Zweibel, "On National Healthcare Decisions Day: Foundation Reflections on Efforts to Promote End-of-Life Planning," *GrantWatch*, *Healthaffairs.org*, April 16, 2013, http://healthaffairs.org/blog/ 2013/04/16/on-national-healthcare-decisions-day-foundation-reflections-on-efforts-to-promote-end-of-life-planning/?cat=grantwatch.

34. Ibid.

EPILOGUE

1. Sidney M. Wolfe, Cynthia Williams, and Alex Zaslow, "Public Citizen's Health Research Group Ranking of the Rate of State Medical Boards' Serious Disciplinary Actions, 2009–2011," Public Citizen, last modified May 17, 2012, http://www.citizen.org/documents/2034.pdf.

2. George D. Lundberg, *Severed Trust* (New York: Basic Books/Perseus, 2000), 74.

BIBLIOGRAPHY

Agency for Healthcare Research and Quality. "Addressing Racial and Ethnic Disparities in Health Care." Last modified April 2013. http://www.ahrq.gov/research/findings/factsheets/minority/disparit/.

Alpha Omega Alpha Honor Medical Society. Last modified 2013. http://www.alphaomegaalpha.org/.

Altman, Lawrence K. "Big Doses of Chemotherapy Drug Killed Patient, Hurt 2d." *New York Times*, March 24, 1995: A18. Available online. http://www.nytimes.com/1995/03/24/us/big-doses-of-chemotherapy-drug-killed-patient-hurt-2d.html.

American Academy of Family Physicians. Last modified 2013. http://www.aafp.org/home.html.

American Psychological Association. "Ray's Race: Running Psychologists Presents the 34th Annual Ray's Race 5K Run and Walk." Last modified May 2012. www.apa.org/about/division/officers/dialogue/2012/05/rays-race.aspx.

Anderson, Gerard F., Uwe E. Reinhardt, Peter S. Hussey, and Varduhi Petrosyan. "It's the Prices, Stupid: Why the United States Is So Different from Other Countries." *Health Affairs* 22, no. 3 (2003): 89–105. doi:10.1377/hlthaff.22.3.89.

Andrews, Michelle. "Questions Arise about Robotic Surgery's Cost, Effectiveness." *Kaiser Health News*. April 23, 2013. http://www.kaiserhealthnews.org/features/insuring-your-health/2013/042313-michelle-andrews-robotic-surgery.aspx.

Andrzejczak, Olivia Victoria. "60 Minutes' Ace's Death Echoes of His Own Investigations." *Houston Chronicle*, July 30, 2009. http://www.chron.com/news/article/60-Minutes-ace-s-death-echoes-his-own-1747718.php.

———. "Lawsuit: TV Producer Pumped Full of Drugs." Timesunion.com, August 9, 2009.

Angell, Marcia. "Excess in the Pharmaceutical Industry." *Canadian Medical Association Journal* 171, no. 12 (December 7, 2004): 1451–53. doi:10.1503/cmaj.1041594.

"Another Alleged Drug Kickback Scheme." *New York Times*, April 27, 2013. http://www.nytimes.com/2013/04/28/opinion/sunday/another-alleged-drug-kickback-scheme.html.

Association for Molecular Pathology et al. v. Myriad Genetics, Inc. et al. 569 U.S. 12-398 (2013). http://www.law.cornell.edu/supremecourt/text/12-398-writing-12-398_SYLLABUS.

Babcock, Charles. "Data on Hospital Errors to Be Deleted." *Boston Globe,* May 3, 2013. http://www.bostonglobe.com/news/nation/2013/05/02/delete-data-life-threatening-hospital-mistakes-from-website/LkVNaa9CKBlQmMIwODdvWI/story.html.

Banks, James, and James Smith. "International Comparisons in Health Economics." RAND Corporation. Last modified October 2011. http://www.rand.org/content/dam/rand/pubs/working_papers/2011/RAND_WR880.pdf.

Barbash, Gabriel I., and Sherry A. Glied. "New Technology and Health Care Costs: The Case of Robot-Assisted Surgery." *New England Journal of Medicine* 363 (2010): 701–4. doi:10.1056/NEJMp1006602.

Bernstein, Nina. "How to Charge $546 for Six Liters of Saltwater." *New York Times*, August 25, 2013. http://www.nytimes.com/2013/08/27/health/exploring-salines-secret-costs.html.

Berwick, Donald M. "Controlling Variation in Health Care: A Consultation from Walter Shewhart." *Medical Care* 29, no. 12 (December 1991): 1212–25.

"Best Grad Schools." Special Issue, *U.S. News & World Report* 2014: D-95–D-105. http://grad-schools.usnews.rankingsandreviews.com/best-graduate-schools.

Bezruchka, Stephen. "Culture and Medicine: Is Globalization Dangerous to Our Health?" *Western Journal of Medicine* 172, no. 5 (2000): 332–34. doi:10.1377/hlthaff.2012.0357.

Bleich, Sara. "Medical Errors: Five Years after the IOM Report." Commonwealth Fund. Last modified July 2005. http://www.commonwealthfund.org/usr_doc/830_bleich_errors.pdf.

Bogdanich, Walt. "Viewpoint." *Leifer Report* (Spring 1992): 6–7.

Boisaubin, E. V., and R. E. Levine. "Identifying and Assisting the Impaired Physician." *American Journal of Medical Sciences* 322, no. 1 (July 2001): 31–36. http://www.ncbi.nlm.nih.gov/pubmed/11465244.

Bomey, Nathan. "University of Michigan Wellness Pioneer Dee Edington Launches Start-up." *Ann Arbor News*, October 23, 2012. http://www.annarbor.com/business-review/university-of-michigan-wellness-pioneer-dee-edington-launches-startup/.

Bonifield, John. "Ohio Family: Hospital 'Botched' Transplant, Threw Out Kidney." CNN, August 30, 2013. http://www.cnn.com/2013/08/30/health/transplant-kidney-thrown-away/.

Boodman, Sandra G. "The Pain of Wrong Site Surgery." *Washington Post*, June 20, 2011. http://articles.washingtonpost.com/2011-06-20/national/35235752_1_wrong-site-surgery-wrong-site-surgery-universal-protocol.

Bornstein, David. "Medicine's Search for Meaning." *New York Times Opinionator*, September 18, 2013. http://opinionator.blogs.nytimes.com/2013/09/18/medicines-search-for-meaning/.

Brawley, Otis W. *How We Do Harm: A Doctor Breaks Ranks about Being Sick in America.* New York: St. Martin's Press, 2011.

Brill, Steven. "Bitter Pill: How Outrageous Pricing and Egregious Profits Are Destroying Health Care." *Time*, March 4, 2013: 16–55. https://www.scrollkit.com/s/BaSaTCZ.

Brownlee, Shannon, John E. Wennberg, Michael J. Barry, Elliott S. Fisher, Julie P. W. Bynum, and David C. Goodman. Edited by Kristen K. Bronner. *Improving Patient Decision-Making in Health Care: A 2012 Dartmouth Atlas Report Highlighting the New England Region.* The Dartmouth Institute for Health Policy & Clinical Practice, November 29, 2012. http://www.dartmouthatlas.org/downloads/reports/01_Decision_Making_New_England_Region.pdf.

Byock, Ira. *Dying Well.* New York: Riverhead, 1997.

Caba, Justin. "Texas Mom's Cancer Misdiagnosis: 54-Year-Old Herlinda Garcia Suffered 7 Months of Chemo, Damages Included Depression and Anxiety." *Medical Daily*, July 17, 2013. http://www.medicaldaily.com/texas-moms-cancer-misdiagnosis-54-year-old-herlinda-garcia-suffered-7-months-chemo-damages-included.

Calikoglu, Sule, Robert Murray, and Dianne Feeney. "Hospital Pay-for-Performance Programs in Maryland Produced Strong Results, Including Reduced Hospital-Acquired Conditions." *Health Affairs* 31, no. 12 (December 2012): 2649–58. doi:10.1377/hlthaff.2012.0357.

"Cancer Patient Tells of Rips in Health Insurance Safety Net." CNN.com, June 16, 2009. http://www.cnn.com/2009/POLITICS/06/16/health.care.hearing/.

Cappiello, Elizabeth J. "Physician Payment Sunshine Act." *Health Law Alert News Letter* 2 (2010). Ober Kaler Attorneys at Law. Last modified 2010. http://www.ober.com/publications/1101-physician-payment-sunshine-act.

"Care of Chronic Illness in the Last Two Years of Life." Dartmouth Atlas of Health Care. Last modified 2013. http://www.dartmouthatlas.org/data/topic/topic.aspx?cat=1.

Carrns, Ann. "Deciding When to Enter a Palliative Care Unit." *New York Times*, September 4, 2013. http://www.nytimes.com/2013/09/04/your-money/deciding-when-to-enter-a-palliative-care-unit.html.

Cass, Connie, and Ricardo Alonso-Zaldivar. "What Now? Q & A about Latest Snag in Health Care Law." *Associated Press*, July 4, 2013. http://bigstory.ap.org/article/what-now-qa-about-latest-snag-health-care-law.

Cassell, Christine K. "The Patient-Physician Covenant: An Affirmation of Asklepios." *Annals of Internal Medicine* 60, no. 5 (March 15, 1996): 291–93. http://www.ncbi.nlm.nih.gov/pubmed/8998907.

Catalyst for Payment Reform and Health Care Incentives Improvement Institute. *Report Card on State Price Transparency Laws*. Health Care Incentives, March 18, 2013. http://www.hci3.org/sites/default/files/files/Report_PriceTransLaws_114.pdf.

Centers for Disease Control and Prevention. "Chronic Diseases and Health Promotion." Last modified August 13, 2012. http://www.cdc.gov/chronicdisease/overview/index.htm.

———. "Fast Facts: Smoking and Tobacco Use." Last modified 2013. http://www.cdc.gov/tobacco/data_statistics/fact_sheets/fast_facts/.

———. "FASTSTATS: Health Insurance Coverage." Last modified August 20, 2012. http://www.cdc.gov/nchs/fastats/hinsure.htm.

———. "A Framework for Patient-Centered Health Risk Assessments." Last modified December 12, 2011. http://www.cdc.gov/policy/opth/hra/.

———. *Health, United States, 2011: With Special Feature on Socioeconomic Status and Health*. National Center for Health Statistics: Hyattsville, Md., 2011. http://www.cdc.gov/nchs/data/hus/hus11.pdf.

Centers for Medicare and Medicaid Services. "National Health Expenditure Projections 2011–2021." http://www.cms.gov/Research-Statistics-Data-and-Systems/Statistics-Trends-and-Reports/NationalHealthExpendData/Downloads/Proj2011PDF.pdf.

———. "National Health Expenditures: 2011 Highlights." http://www.cms.gov/Research-Statistics-Data-and-Systems/Statistics-Trends-and-Reports/NationalHealthExpendData/Downloads/highlights.pdf

"CEO Compensation, 2012." *Forbes*. Last modified December 2012. http://www.forbes.com/lists.

Chen, Pauline W. "For Med Students, Love from the Drug Rep." *Well*, October 3, 2013. http://well.blogs.nytimes.com/2013/10/03/for-med-students-love-from-the-drug-rep/.

Cohen, Phil. "Deming's 14 Points." HCi. http://www.hci.com.au/hcisite2/articles/deming.htm.

Colella, Giovanni. "To Bring Healthcare Prices Down, Consumers Must Demand Price Transparency." *Forbes*, March 20, 2013. http://www.forbes.com/sites/realspin/2013/03/20/to-bring-healthcare-prices-down-consumers-must-demand-price-transparency/.

Collins, G. "Frankenstein Goes to Congress." *New York Times*, October 4, 2013. http://www.nytimes.com/2013/10/05/opinion/collins-frankenstein-goes-to-congress.html.

Collins, S. R., and Karen Davis. "Transparency in Health Care: The Time Has Come." Commonwealth Fund. Last modified March 15, 2006. http://www.commonwealthfund.org/Publications/Testimonies/2006/Mar/Transparency-in-Health-Care--The-Time-Has-Come.aspx.

Collins, S. R., Ruth Robertson, Tracy Garber, and Michelle M. Doty. "Insuring the Future: Current Trends in Health Coverage and the Effects of Implementing the Affordable Care Act." Commonwealth Fund. Last modified April 2013. http://www.commonwealthfund.org/~/media/Files/Publications/Fund Report/2013/Apr/1681_Collins_insuring_future_biennial_survey_2012_FINAL.pdf.

Committee on Quality of Health Care in America and Institute of Medicine. *Crossing the Quality Chasm: A New Health System for the 21st Century*. Washington, D.C.: National Academy Press, 2001.

Commonwealth Fund. *Transparency in Health Care: The Time Has Come*. New York: The Commonwealth Fund, March 15, 2006. http://www.commonwealthfund.org/Publications/Testimonies/2006/Mar/Transparency-in-Health-Care--The-Time-Has-Come.aspx.

Conaboy, Chelsea. "Report: Variations in Quality of Care a 'Hidden' Curriculum for New Doctors at Teaching Hospitals." *Boston Globe*, October 30, 2012. http://www.boston.com/whitecoatnotes/2012/10/30/report-variations-quality-care-hidden-curriculum-for-new-doctors-teaching-hospitals/CGdrLdXtCgy3qFJwhi7t9I/story.html.

Creswell, Julie, and Reed Abelson. "New Laws and Rising Costs Create a Surge in Supersizing Hospitals." *New York Times*, August 12, 2013. http://www.nytimes.com/2013/08/13/business/bigger-hospitals-may-lead-to-bigger-bills-for-patients.html.

Daly, Rich. "CMS Data Show Wide Variation in Hospital Billing." *Modern Healthcare*. Last modified May 8, 2013. http://www.modernhealthcare.com/article/20130508/NEWS/305089960#.

Damman, Olga C., Michelle Hendriks, Jany Rademakers, Diana M. J. Delnoij, and Peter P. Groenewegen. "How Do Healthcare Consumers Process and Evaluate Comparative Healthcare Information? A Qualitative Study Using Cognitive Interviews." *BMC Public Health* 9, no. 423 (2009): 423. doi:10.1186/1471-2458-9-423.

"Dangerous Supplements: What You Don't Know about These 12 Supplements Could Hurt You." *Consumer Reports*. Last modified May 2012. http://www.consumerreports.org/cro/2012/05/dangerous-supplements/.

Dartmouth Institute for Health Policy and Clinical Practice. "Q & A with Dr. Jack Wennberg: What's Wrong with the U.S. Health-Care System?" Last modified March 21, 2008. http://www.dartmouthatlas.org/downloads/press/Wennberg_interviews_DartMed.pdf.

Davis, D. A., Paul E. Mazmanian, Michael Fordis, R. Van Harrison, Kevin E. Thorpe, and Laure Perrier. "Accuracy of Physician Self-Assessment Compared with Observed Measures of Competence: A Systematic Review." *Journal of the American Medical Association* 296, no. 9 (September 6, 2006): 1094–1102. doi:10.1001/jama.296.9.1094.

Davis, Karen, Cathy Schoen, and Kristof Stremikis. *Mirror, Mirror on the Wall: How the Performance of the U.S. Health Care System Compares Internationally*. New York: Commonwealth Foundation, 2010. http://www.commonwealthfund.org/~/media/Files/Publications/Fund Report/2010/Jun/1400_Davis_Mirror_Mirror_on_the_wall_2010.pdf.

Department for Professional Employees AFL-CIO. "2012 Fact Sheet: The U.S. Health Care System: An International Perspective." Last modified April 2012. http://dpeaflcio.org/wp-content/uploads/US-Health-Care-in-Intl-Perspective-2012.pdf.

Docteur, Elizabeth, and Robert A. Berenson. *How Does the Quality of U.S. Health Care Compare Internationally? Timely Analysis of Immediate Health Policy Issues*. Robert Wood Johnson Foundation, August 2009. http://www.urban.org/uploadedpdf/411947_ushealthcare_quality.pdf.

"Doctor Who Cut Off Wrong Leg Is Defended by Colleagues." *New York Times*, September 17, 1995. http://www.nytimes.com/1995/09/17/us/doctor-who-cut-off-wrong-leg-is-defended-by-colleagues.html.

Douthat, Russ. "Obamacare, Failing Ahead of Schedule." *New York Times*, October 19, 2013. http://www.nytimes.com/2013/10/20/opinion/sunday/douthat-obamacare-failing-ahead-of-schedule.html.

Doyle, Jim. "Blunders: Botched Brain Surgery Prompts Extensive Review at SSM Health' Care." *St. Louis Post Dispatch*, May 5, 2013. http://www.stltoday.com/business/local/botched-brain-surgery-prompts-extensive-review-at-ssm-health-care/article_df1f66b8-ba03-5ba1-8e93-ce0cc771f0a5.html.

Dychtwald, Ken, and Joe Flower. *Age Wave: How the Most Important Trend of Our Time Can Change Your Future*. New York: Bantam, 1990.

Elias, Peter. "Sunday Dialogue: Handling Medical Errors." *New York Times*, October 18, 2013. http://www.nytimes.com/2013/10/20/opinion/sunday/sunday-dialogue-handling-medical-errors.html.

Enthoven, Alain C., and Laura A. Tollen. "Competition in Health Care: It Takes Systems to Pursue Quality and Efficiency." *Health Affairs* (September 7, 2005): 420–33. doi:10.1377/hlthaff.w5.420.

Epstein, Ronald M., and Edward M. Hundert. "Defining and Assessing Professional Competence." *Journal of the American Medical Association* 287, no. 2 (January 9, 2002): 226–35. doi:10.1001/jama.287.2.226.

Fahrenthold, Laura A. "4-yr.-old Dies after Surgery." *New York Daily News*, March 23, 1995. http://www.nydailynews.com/archives/news/4-yr-old-dies-surgery-article-1.688316.

Families USA. "Resources for Consumers." Last modified July 2011. http://www.familiesusa.org/resources/resources-for-consumers/.

Farrell, Diana, Eric Jensen, Bob Kocher, Nick Lovegrove, Fareed Melhem, Lenny Mendonca, and Beth Parish. *Accounting for the Cost of U.S. Health Care: A New Look at Why Americans Spend More*. McKinsey Global Institute. December 2008. http://www.mckinsey.com/insights/health_systems_and_services/accounting_for_the_cost_of_us_health_care.

Field, Marilyn J., and Christine K. Cassell. *Approaching Death: Improving Care at the End of Life*. Washington, D.C.: National Academy Press, 1997.

Fisher, Nicole. "Closing Racial and Ethnic Disparity Gaps: Implications of the Affordable Care Act," *Forbes*. Last modified May 28, 2013. http://www.forbes.com/sites/theapothecary/2013/05/28/closing-racial-and-ethnic-disparity-gaps-implications-of-the-affordable-care-act/.

FoxNews.com. "Cancer-Free Woman Undergoes 7 Months of Chemotherapy after Misdiagnosis." July 18, 2013. http://www.foxnews.com/health/2013/07/18/cancer-free-woman-undergoes-7-months-chemotherapy-after-misdiagnosis/.

Frech, H. E., Stephen T. Parente, and John Hoff. "US Health Care: A Reality Check on Cross-Country Comparisons." AEI. Last modified July 11, 2012. http://www.aei.org/outlook/health/global-health/us-health-care-a-reality-check-on-cross-country-comparisons.

Frier, Sarah. "Insurers Profit from Health Law They Fought Against." Bloomberg. Last modified January 5, 2012. http://www.bloomberg.com/news/2012-01-05/health-insurer-profit-rises-as-obama-s-health-law-supplies-revenue-boost.html.

Fries, James F. "Aging, Natural Death, and the Compression of Morbidity." *New England Journal of Medicine* 303 (July 17, 1980): 130–35. doi:10.1056/NEJM198007173030304.

Frost, Robert. "The Road Not Taken." Available online at http://www.poetryfoundation.org/poem/173536.

Garver, Rob, and Charles Seife. "Double Dose: In Second Case of Flawed Drug Research, FDA Response Was Slow and Secretive." ProPublica. Last modified April 17, 2013. http://www.propublica.org/article/double-dose-in-second-case-of-flawed-drug-research-fda-response-was-slow.

———. "FDA Lets Drugs Approved on Fraudulent Research Stay on the Market." ProPublica. Last modified April 15, 2013. http://www.propublica.org/article/fda-let-drugs-approved-on-fraudulent-research-stay-on-the-market.

Gawande, Atul. *BETTER: A Surgeon's Notes on Performance*. New York: Henry Holt, 2007.

———. "The Cost Conundrum." *New Yorker*, June 1, 2009. http://www.newyorker.com/reporting/2009/06/01/090601fa_fact_gawande.

Gertz, Matt. "Nets Ignore Testimony of Cancer Patient Denied Coverage by Insurer." Media Matters, June 22, 2009. http://mediamatters.org/research/2009/06/22/nets-ignore-testimony-of-cancer-patient-denied/151406.

Ghaferi, Amir A., John D. Birkmeyer, and Justin B. Dimick. "Variation in Hospital Mortality Associated with Inpatient Surgery." *New England Journal of Medicine* 361 (October 1, 2009): 1368–75. doi:10.1056/NEJMsa0903048.

Gibbons, Luz, José M. Belizán, Jeremy A. Lauer, Ana P. Betrán, Mario Merialdi, and Fernando Althabe. "The Global Numbers and Costs of Additionally Needed and Unnecessary Caesarean Sections Performed per Year: Overuse as a Barrier to Universal Coverage." World Health Organization. Last modified 2010. http://www.who.int/healthsystems/topics/financing/healthreport/30C-sectioncosts.pdf.

Ginsburg, Jack A., Robert B. Doherty, J. Fred Ralston Jr., and Naomi Senkeeto. "Achieving a High Performance Health Care System with Universal Access: What the United States Can Learn from Other Countries." *Annals of Internal Medicine* 148, no. 1 (2008): 55–75. doi:10.7326/0003-4819-148-1-200801010-00196.

Goldacre, Ben. "Trial sans Error: How Pharma-Funded Research Cherry-Picks Positive Results [Excerpt]." *Scientific American*, February 13, 2013. http://www.

scientificamerican.com/article.cfm?id=trial-sans-error-how-pharma-funded-research-cherry-picks-positive-results.

Goodnough, Abby. "As Nurse Lay Dying, Offering Herself as Instruction in Caring." *New York Times*, January 10, 2013. http://www.nytimes.com/2013/01/11/us/fatally-ill-and-making-herself-the-lesson.html.

Gorman, Christine. "The Disturbing Case of the Cure that Killed the Patient." *Time*, April 3, 1995. http://content.time.com/time/magazine/article/0,9171,982768,00.html.

Grady, Denise. "Hospitals Profit from Surgical Errors, Study Finds." *New York Times*, April 17, 2013. http://www.nytimes.com/2013/04/17/health/hospitals-profit-from-surgical-errors-study-finds.html.

Griffin, Drew, and David Fitzpatrick. "US Patients Try Stem Cell Therapies Abroad," CNN.com, June 2, 2009. http://www.cnn.com/2009/HEALTH/06/02/stem.cell.therapy/.

"Guru: W. Edwards Deming." *Economist*. Last modified June 5, 2009. http://www.economist.com/node/13805735.

Hadler, Nortin M. *The Last Well Person: How to Stay Well Despite the Health Care System.* Montreal: McGill Queen's University Press, 2004.

Hancock, Jay. "Health Insurance Actuaries in the Hot Seat On 'Rate Shock.'" *Kaiser Health News*, April 13, 2013. http://www.kaiserhealthnews.org/stories/2013/april/18/actuaries-ties-to-insurance-rate-shock.aspx.

Harris, Gardiner. "Doctor Faces Suits over Cardiac Stents." *New York Times*, December 5, 2010. http://www.nytimes.com/2010/12/06/health/06stent.html.

Health Care for America Now. "Health Insurance Industry." http://healthcareforamericanow.org/ourissues/health-insurance-industry/.

Health Care Incentives Improvement Institute (HCI3). "Affordability of Health Care: Metrics for Tranformation." Last modified 2012. http://www.hci3.org/content/affordability-health-care-metrics-transformation.

Hildebrand, Janet S., Susan M. Gapstur, Peter T. Campbell, Mia M. Gaudet, and Alpa V. Patel. "Recreational Physical Activity and Leisure-Time Sitting in Relation to Postmenopausal Breast Cancer Risk." *Cancer Epidemiology, Biomarkers & Prevention*, October 22, 2013. doi: 10.1158/1055-9965.EPI-13-0407.

Hunt, Vivian, Nigel Manson, and Paul Morgan. "A Wake-Up Call for Big Pharma." McKinsey & Company. Last modified December 2011. http://www.mckinsey.com/insights/health_systems/a_wake-up_call_for_big_pharma.

Institute of Medicine of the National Academies. *U.S. Health in International Perspective: Shorter Lives, Poorer Health*. Washington, D.C.: National Academies Press, 2012. http://www.nap.edu/openbook.php?record_id=13497.

Intermountain Health Care. Last modified 2013. http://intermountainhealthcare.org/providers/specialties.html.

International Federation of Health Plans. *International Federation of Health Plans: 2012 Comparative Price Report; Variation in Medical and Hospital Prices by Country.* 2012. http://hushp.harvard.edu/sites/default/files/downloadable_files/IFHP 2012 Comparative Price Report.pdf.

James, Brent C., and Elizabeth H. Hammond. "The Challenge of Variation in Medical Practice." *Archive of Pathology and Laboratory Medicine* 124, no. 7 (July 2000): 1001–3. http://www.ncbi.nlm.nih.gov/pubmed/10888775.

James, Susan Donaldson. "Toledo Hospital Threw Out Donor Kidney, Now Denies Negligence." ABCNews, August 29, 2013. http://abcnews.go.com/Health/toledo-hospital-threw-donor-kidney-now-denies-negligence/story?id=20110334.

Janicki, Hubert. "Employment-Based Health Insurance: 2010." United States Census Bureau/U.S. Department of Commerce. Last modified February 2013. http://www.census.gov/prod/2013pubs/p70-134.pdf.

Kaiser Family Foundation. "Employer Health Benefits 2010 Summary of Findings." September 2010.

———. "The Uninsured and the Difference Health Insurance Makes." September 1, 2012. http://kff.org/uninsured/fact-sheet/the-uninsured-and-the-difference-health-insurance/.

Kaiser Family Foundation and Health Research and Educational Trust. "Employer Health Benefits: 2012 Annual Survey." Last modified September 11, 2012. http:// kaiserfamilyfoundation.files.wordpress.com/2013/03/8345-employer-health-benefits-annual-survey-full-report-0912.pdf.

Kane, Jason. "Health Costs: How the U.S. Compares with Other Countries." *The Rundown*, PBS NewsHour, October 22, 2012. http://www.pbs.org/newshour/rundown/2012/10/ health-costs-how-the-us-compares-with-other-countries.html.

Katz, Dana, Arthur L. Caplan, and Jon F. Merz. "All Gifts Large and Small." *American Journal of Bioethics* 3, no. 3 (Summer 2003): 39–46. Available online at http://repository. upenn.edu/cgi/viewcontent.cgi?article=1050&context=bioethics_papers.

Keckley, Paul H. *2011 Survey of Health Care Consumers Global Report*. Deloitte. 2011. http://www.deloitte.com/assets/dcom-unitedstates/localassets/documents/us_chs_ 2011consumersurveyglobal_062111.pdf.

———. *Deloitte 2012 Survey of U.S. Health Care Consumers: The Performance of the Health Care System and Health Care Reform*. Deloitte. 2012. http://www.deloitte.com/ assets/dcom-unitedstates/localassets/documents/healthreformissues   briefs/us_chs_ issuebrief_2012consumersurvey_061212.pdf.

———. *Health Care Price Transparency: A Strategic Perspective for State Government Leaders*. Washington, D.C.: Deloitte, 2007. http://www.essisystems.com/research/Health_ Care_Price_Transparency.pdf.

Kim, Theodore, and Tammy Webber. "Third Baby Dies after Error at Indiana Hospital." *USA Today*, September 20, 2006. http://usatoday30.usatoday.com/news/nation/2006-09-20-baby-deaths_x.htm.

Klein, Ezra. "Health-Insurance Industry: Still Not That Profitable." *Washington Post*, February 24, 2011. http://voices.washingtonpost.com/ezra-klein/2011/02/health-insurance_ industry_stil.html.

———. "Why an MRI Costs $1,080 in America and $280 in France." *Wonkblog, Washington Post*, March 3, 2012. http://www.washingtonpost.com/blogs/wonkblog/post/why-an-mri-costs-1080-in-america-and-280-in-france/2011/08/25/gIQAVHztoR_blog.html.

Kohn, Linda T., Janet M. Corrigan, and Molla S. Donaldson. *To Err Is Human: Building a Safer Health Care System*. Washington, D.C.: National Academy Press, 2000.

Korenstein, D., A. S. Keyhani, and S. Ross. "Physician Attitudes toward Industry: A View across the Specialties." *Archives of Surgery* 145, no. 6 (June 2010): 570–77. doi:10.1001/ archsurg.2010.75.

Kornfield, Rachel, Julie Donohue, Ernst. R. Berndt, and G. Caleb Alexander. "Promotion of Prescription Drugs to Consumer and Providers, 2001–2010." *PLOS ONE* 8, no. 3 (March 4, 2013). http://www.plosone.org/article/info%3Adoi%2F10.1371%2Fjournal.pone. 0055504.

Kotz, Deborah. "Maternity Hospitals Push to Reduce C-Section Rate and Medical Interventions." Boston.com, October 7, 2012. http://www.boston.com/lifestyle/health/2012/10/14/ maternity-hospitals-push-reduce-section-rate-and-medical-interventions/ UM95Mb3oO1lLmcT0Ql4II6H/singlepage.html.

Krans, Brian. "Why Do We Get So Little Value from the Healthcare System?" *Healthline-News*, April 18, 2013. http://www.healthline.com/health-news/policy-why-is-healthcare-so-over-priced-041813.

Kübler-Ross, Elisabeth. *On Death and Dying*. New York: Macmillan Publishing, 1969.

LaFleur, J. T., Weber, C. Ornstein, and J. Larson. "How We Analyzed Medicare's Drug Data." ProPublica, May 11, 2013. http://www.propublica.org/article/how-we-analyzed-medicares-drug-data-long-methodology.

Lundberg, George D. *Severed Trust*. New York: Basic Books/Perseus, 2000.

MacDorman, Marian F., Donna L. Hoyert, and T. J. Matthews. "Recent Declines in Infant Mortality in the United States, 2005–2011." *NCHS Data Brief*, no. 120 (April 2013). http:/ /www.cdc.gov/nchs/data/databriefs/db120.pdf.

Mahar, Maggie. "Braveheart." *Dartmouth Medicine* (Winter 2007). http://dartmed. dartmouth.edu/winter07/html/braveheart.php.

Mahler, Jonathan. "The Antidepressant Dilemma," *New York Times*, November 21, 2004. http://www.nytimes.com/2004/11/21/magazine/21TEENS.html?pagewanted=all& position=&_r=0.

Makary, Marty. *Unaccountable: What Hospitals Won't Tell You and How Transparency Can Revolutionize Health Care*. New York: Bloomsbury Press, 2012.

Martin, Anne, David Lassman, Benjamin Washington, Aaron Catlin, and the National Health Expenditure Accounts Team. "Growth in US Health Spending Remained Slow in 2010; Health Share of Gross Domestic Product Was Unchanged from 2009." *Health Affairs* 31, no. 1 (January 2012): 1–13. doi:10.1377/hlthaff.2011.1135.

Martinez, Michael E., and Robin A. Cohen. "Health Insurance Coverage: Early Release of Estimates from the National Health Interview Survey, January–September 2012." Centers for Disease Control. Last modified March 2013. http://www.cdc.gov/nchs/data/nhis/earlyrelease/Insur201303.pdf.

Marwah, Sanjay, and Sham Lal Singla. "Spirit-Induced Cautery Burns: An Unusual Iatrogenic Injury." *Internet Journal of Surgery* 22, no. 2 (2010), http://ispub.com/IJS/22/2/9414.

"Mass General Hospital Ranked No. 1." Harvard Medical School. July 17, 2012, http://hms.harvard.edu/news/mass-general-hospital-ranked-no-1-7-17-12.

McFadden, D. W., E. Calvario, and C. Graves. "The Devil Is in the Details: The Pharmaceutical Industry's Use of Gifts to Physicians as Marketing Strategy." *Journal of Surgical Research* 140, no. 1 (June 1, 2007): 1–5. http://www.ncbi.nlm.nih.gov/pubmed/17481979.

McGinnis, J. Michael, LeighAnne Olsen, Katharine Bothner, Daniel O'Neill, and Dara Aisner. *Learning What Works Best: The Nation's Need for Evidence on Comparative Effectiveness in Health Care*. Washington, D.C.: Institute of Medicine, 2007. http://www.ncbi.nlm.nih.gov/books/NBK64784/.

McNaughton-Collins, Mary F., and Michael J. Barry. "One Man at a Time: Resolving the PSA Controversy." *New England Journal of Medicine* 365 (2011): 1951–53. doi:10.1056/NEJMp1111894.

Medicare.gov. "How Do I File an Appeal?" http://www.medicare.gov/claims-and-appeals/file-an-appeal/appeals.html.

Mehta, Sonya P., Sanjay M. Bhananker, Karen L. Posner, and Karen B. Domino. "Operating Room Fires: A Closed Claims Analysis." *Anesthesiology* 118, no. 5: 1133-39. doi: 10.1097/ALN.0b013e31828afa7b.

Menacker, Fay, and Brady E. Hamilton. "Recent Trends in Cesarean Delivery in the United States." Centers for Disease Control, *NCHS Data Brief*, no. 35 (March 2010). http://www.cdc.gov/nchs/data/databriefs/db35.htm.

Millenson, Michael L. *Demanding Medical Excellence*. Chicago: University of Chicago Press, 1997.

Milstein, Arnold, and Nancy E. Adler. "Out of Sight, Out of Mind: Why Doesn't Widespread Clinical Quality Failure Command Our Attention?" *Health Affairs* 22, no. 2 (2003): 119–27. http://www.ncbi.nlm.nih.gov/pubmed/12674415.

Mintzes, Barbara, Morris L. Barer, Richard L. Kravitz, Ken Bassett, Joel Lexchin, Arminée Kazanjian, Robert G. Evans, Richard Pan, and Stephen A. Marion. "How Does Direct-to-Consumer Advertising (DTCA) Affect Prescribing? A Survey in Primary Care Environments with and without Legal DTCA." *Canadian Medical Association Journal* 169, no. 5 (September 2, 2003): 405–12. http://www.ncbi.nlm.nih.gov/pmc/articles/PMC183290/.

Mitchell, Russ. "29 States Get 'F' for Price Transparency Laws." *Capsules: The KHN Blog*, *Kaiserhealthnews.org*, March 18, 2013. http://capsules.kaiserhealthnews.org/?p=17815.

National Association of Public Hospitals and Health Systems. "History of Public Hospitals and Health Systems." Last modified 2013. http://www.naph.org/Homepage-Sections/Explore/History.aspx.

National Cancer Institute. "FDA Approval for Bevacizumab." http://www.cancer.gov/cancertopics/druginfo/fda-bevacizumab.

Neuman, Jennifer, Deborah Korenstein, Joseph S. Ross, and Salomeh Keyhani. "Prevalence of Financial Conflicts of Interest among Panel Members Producing Clinical Practice Guidelines in Canada and the United States: Cross Sectional Study." *British Medical Journal* 343 (2011): d5621. doi:http://dx.doi.org/10.1136/bmj.d5621.

Newbergh, Carolyn. "The Dartmouth Atlas of Health Care." In *Robert Wood Johnson Foundation Anthology: To Improve Health and Health Care*, edited by Stephen L. Isaacs and James R. Knickman, 25–48. San Francisco: Jossey-Bass, 2006.

Newman, Rick. "Why Health Insurers Make Lousy Villains." *MONEY, USNews.com*, August 25, 2009. http://money.usnews.com/money/blogs/flowchart/2009/08/25/why-health-insurers-make-lousy-villains.

O'Malley, Kate, and Nancy Zweibel. "On National Healthcare Decisions Day: Foundation Reflections on Efforts to Promote End-of-Life Planning." *GrantWatch, Healthaffairs.org*, April 16, 2013. http://healthaffairs.org/blog/2013/04/16/on-national-healthcare-decisions-day-foundation-reflections-on-efforts-to-promote-end-of-life-planning/?cat=grantwatch.

Open Secrets.org, Center for Responsive Politics. "Lobbying: Pharmaceuticals/Health Products." Last modified 2013. http://www.opensecrets.org/lobby/indusclient.php?id=H04.

Organisation for Economic Development and Cooperation. "OECD Health Data 2010: How Does Canada Compare?" June 29, 2010. http://www.oecd.org/els/health-systems/Briefing-Note-CANADA-2013.pdf.

———. "OECD Health Data 2010: How Does Germany Compare." June 29, 2010.

———. "OECD Health Data 2010: How Does Spain Compare." June 29, 2010.

———. "OECD Health Data 2010: How Does Sweden Compare." June 29, 2010.

———. "OECD Health Data 2011: How Does the United States Compare." June 29.

———. "OECD Health Data 2012: How Does the United States Compare."

Pear, Robert. "A Limit on Consumer Costs Is Delayed in Health Care Law." *New York Times*, August 12, 2013. http://www.nytimes.com/2013/08/13/us/a-limit-on-consumer-costs-is-delayed-in-health-care-law.html.

Pennsylvania Health Care Cost Containment Council. "Pennsylvania Health Care Cost Containment Council." Last modified 2013. www.phc4.org.

Peterson, Christopher, and Martin Seligman. *Character Strengths and Virtues*. Oxford: Oxford University Press, 2004.

Pollack, Andrew. "Doctors Denounce Cancer Drug Prices of $100,000 a Year." *New York Times*, April 25, 2013. http://www.nytimes.com/2013/04/26/business/cancer-physicians-attack-high-drug-costs.html.

———. "Health Care Costs Climb Moderately, Survey Says." *New York Times*, August 20, 2013. http://www.nytimes.com/2013/08/21/business/survey-finds-modest-rise-in-health-insurance-premiums.html.

———. "Looser Guidelines Issued on Prostate Screening." *New York Times*, May 3, 2013. http://www.nytimes.com/2013/05/04/business/prostate-screening-guidelines-are-loosened.html.

Prescott, Gregg. "Holistic Cancer Research: Rife Machines." Holistic Cancer Research.com. http://holisticcancerresearch.com/holistic-cancer-research-rife-machine.html.

Public Citizen. "The Other Drug War: Big Pharma's 625 Washington Lobbyists." Last modified July 23, 2001. http://www.citizen.org/documents/pharmadrugwar.PDF.

PWC Health Research Institute. *Scoring Healthcare: Navigating Customer Experience Ratings*. 2013.

Rabin, Roni Caryn. "Doctors' Lucrative Industry Ties." *Well*, *New York Times*, May 13, 2013. http://well.blogs.nytimes.com/2013/05/13/doctors-lucrative-industry-ties/.

———. "Salesmen in the Surgical Suite." *New York Times*, March 25, 2103. http://www.nytimes.com/2013/03/26/health/salesmen-in-the-surgical-suite.html.

Ramshaw, Emily, and Ryan Murphy. "Payments to Doctors by Pharmaceutical Companies Raise Conflicts of Interest." *New York Times*, November 24, 2011. http://www.nytimes.com/2011/11/25/us/payments-to-doctors-by-pharmaceutical-companies-raise-issues-of-conflicts.html.

Ratey, John L., with Eric Hagerman. *Spark: The Revolutionary New Science of Exercise and the Brain*. New York: Little, Brown and Company, 2008.

Reid, T. R. *The Healing of America*. New York: Penguin, 2010.

Reinhardt, Uwe E. "U.S. Health Care Prices Are the Elephant in the Room." *Economix*, March 29, 2013. http://economix.blogs.nytimes.com/2013/03/29/u-s-health-care-prices-are-the-elephant-in-the-room/.

Relman, Arnold S. *A Second Opinion*. Cambridge, Mass.: Public Affairs/Perseus Books Group, 2007.

ResidentPhysician. "The Official Rankings of 17 Medical Departments for their Resident Physician." Last modified 1999. http://www.residentphysician.com/.

Robert Wood Johnson Foundation. *Consumer Attitudes on Health Care Costs: Insights from Focus Groups in Four U.S. Cities*. January 2013. http://www.rwjf.org/content/dam/farm/reports/issue_briefs/2013/rwjf403428.

———. *Lessons Learned: Consumer Beliefs and Use of Information about Health Care Cost, Resource Use, and Value*. October 2012. http://www.rwjf.org/content/dam/farm/reports/issue_briefs/2012/rwjf402126.

Rosenthal, Elisabeth. "A Push to Sell Testosterone Gels Troubles Doctors." *New York Times*, October 15, 2013. http://www.nytimes.com/2013/10/16/us/a-push-to-sell-testosterone-gels-troubles-doctors.html.

"Saint Luke's Health System CEO Hastings Will Retire." *Kansas City Business Journal*, January 12, 2011. http://www.bizjournals.com/kansascity/news/2011/01/12/saint-lukes-health-system-ceo.html.

Schoen, Cathy, Jacob Lippa, Sara Collins, and David Radley. "State Trends in Premiums and Deductibles, 2003–2011: Eroding Protection and Rising Costs Underscore Need for Action." Commonwealth Fund. Last modified December 2012. http://www.commonwealthfund.org/Publications/Issue-Briefs/2012/Dec/State-Trends-in-Premiums-and-Deductibles.aspx.

Schoen, Cathy, Robin Osborn, Michelle M. Doty, David Squires, Jordon Peugh, and Sandra Applebaum. "A Survey of Primary Care Physicians in Eleven Countries, 2009: Perspectives on Care, Costs, and Experiences." *Health Affairs*, Web Exclusive (Nov. 5, 2009): 1171–83. http://content.healthaffairs.org/content/28/6/w1171.full.html.

Shahinian, Vahakn B., Yong-Fang Kuo, and Scott M. Gilbert. "Reimbursement Policy and Androgen-Deprivation Therapy for Prostate Cancer." *New England Journal of Medicine* 363 (November 4, 2010): 1822–32. doi:10.1056/NEJMsa0910784.

Smith, A., K. E. McCarthy, E. Weber, I. S. Cenzer, J. Boscardin, J. Fisher, and K. Covinsky. "Half of Older Americans Seen in Emergency Department in Last Month of Life: Most Admitted to Hospital, and Many Die There." *Health Affairs* 31, no. 7 (May 31, 2013): 1277–85. doi:10.1377/hlthaff.2011.0922.

Sommers, Roseanna, Susan Dorr Goold, Elizabeth A. McGlynn, Steven D. Pearson, and Marion Danis. "Focus Groups Highlight That Many Patients Object to Clinicians' Focusing on Costs." *Health Affairs* 32, no. 2 (2012): 338–46. doi:10.1377/hlthaff.2012.0686.

Squires, David. *Multinational Comparisons of Health Systems Data, 2010*. Commonwealth Fund. 2012. http://www.commonwealthfund.org/Publications/Chartbooks/2011/Jul/Multinational-Comparisons-of-Health-Systems-Data-2010.aspx.

Stein, Letitia. "Desperate Families Turn to Unproven Stem Cell Treatment." *Tampa Bay Times*, May 27, 2011. http://www.tampabay.com/news/health/medicine/desperate-families-turn-to-unproven-stem-cell-treatment/1172182.

Steinbrook, Robert. "Disclosure of Industry Payments to Physicians." *New England Journal of Medicine* 359, no. 6 (August 7, 2008): 559–61. Available online at http://depts.washington.edu/hmcderma/Steinbrook_NEJM-08.pdf.

Stephan, Pam. "Herlinda Garcia Survived Stage 4 Breast Cancer Misdiagnosis." About.com, July 24, 2013. http://breastcancer.about.com/b/2013/07/24/herlinda-garcia-survived-stage-4-breast-cancer-misdiagnosis.htm.

Thomas, Katie. "U.S. Drug Costs Dropped in 2012, but Rises Loom." *New York Times*, March 18, 2013. http://www.nytimes.com/2013/03/19/business/use-of-generics-produces-an-unusual-drop-in-drug-spending.html.

Tompkins, Christopher P., Stuart H. Altman, and Efrat Eilat. "The Precarious Pricing System for Hospital Services." *Health Affairs* 25, no. 1 (January–February 2006): 45–56. doi:10.1377/hlthaff.25.1.45.

Thompson, Derek. "Why Is American Health Care So Ridiculously Expensive?" *Atlantic*, March 27, 2013. http://www.theatlantic.com/business/archive/2013/03/why-is-american-health-care-so-ridiculously-expensive/274425/.

"Total Medicare Reimbursements per Enrollee, by Adjustment Type." Dartmouth Atlas of Health Care. http://www.dartmouthatlas.org/data/map.aspx?ind=225.

Ubel, Peter. "How Price Transparency Could End Up Increasing Health-Care Costs." *Atlantic*, April 2013. http://www.theatlantic.com/health/archive/2013/04/how-price-transparency-could-end-up-increasing-health-care-costs/274534/.

"Understanding of the Efficiency and Effectiveness of the Health Care System." Dartmouth Atlas of Health Care. Last modified 2013. http://www.dartmouthatlas.org/.

U.S. Government Accountability Office. *Higher Use of Costly Prostate Cancer Treatment by Providers Who Self-Refer Warrants Scrutiny*. Washington, D.C.: U.S. Government Accountability Office, 2013. http://www.gao.gov/products/gao-13-525.

"Update on Health Care Reform." *Consumer Reports*. Last modified March 2013. http://www.consumerreports.org/cro/2012/06/update-on-health-care-reform/index.htm.

Vastag, Brian. "Doctors Groups Call for End to UnnecessaryProcedures." *The Checkup*, *Washington Post*, April 4, 2012. http://www.washingtonpost.com/blogs/the-checkup/post/doctors-groups-call-for-end-to-unnecessary-procedures/2012/04/03/gIQAvrDptS_blog.html.

Vogt, Donna U. *CRS Report for Congress: Direct to Consumer Advertising of Prescription Drugs*. Washington, D.C.: Library of Congress, March 25, 2005. Available online at http://www.law.umaryland.edu/marshall/crsreports/crsdocuments/RL3285303252005.pdf.

Walshe, Kiernan, and Stephen M. Shortell. "When Things Go Wrong: How Health Care Organizations Deal with Major Failures." *Health Affairs* 23, no. 3 (May 2004): 103–11. http://content.healthaffairs.org/content/23/3/103.full.

Wazana, Ashley. "Physicians and the Pharmaceutical Industry: Is a Gift Ever Just a Gift?" *Journal of the American Medical Association* 283, no. 3 (January 19, 2000): 373–80. doi:10.1001/jama.283.3.373.

Weber, Tracy, and C. Ornstein. "Why You Should Care about the Drugs Your Doctor Prescribes." ProPublica, July 15, 2013. http://www.propublica.org/article/why-you-should-care-about-the-drugs-your-doctor-prescribes.

Welch, W. Pete, Mark E. Miller, H. Gilbert Welch, Elliott S. Fisher, and John E. Wennberg. "Geographic Variation in Expenditures for Physicians' Services in the United States." *New England Journal of Medicine* 328 (March 4, 1993): 621–27. doi:10.1056/NEJM199303043280906.

Wennberg, John E. "Unwarranted Variations in Healthcare Delivery: Implications for Academic Medical Centers." *British Medical Journal* 325 (October 26, 2002): 961–64. doi:http://dx.doi.org/10.1136/bmj.325.7370.961.

Wennberg, John, and Alan Gittelsohn. "Small Area Variations in Health Care Delivery." *Science* 182, no. 4117 (December 1973): 1102–8. doi:10.1126/science.182.4117.1102.

Wolfe, Sidney M., Cynthia Williams, and Alex Zaslow. "Public Citizen's Health Research Group Ranking of the Rate of State Medical Boards' Serious Disciplinary Actions, 2009–2011." Public Citizen. Last modified May 17, 2012. http://www.citizen.org/documents/2034.pdf.

World Health Organization. "World Health Report 2000: Health Systems; Improving Performance." Geneva: World Health Organization, 2000, 188–91. http://www.who.int/whr/2000/en/annex07_en.pdf. Full report available at http://www.who.int/whr/2000/en/whr00_en.pdf?ua=1.

YahooNews. "The Sky-High Price of Chemotherapy: Why Do Cancer Drugs Cost So Much?" Last modified May 9, 2013. http://news.yahoo.com/sky-high-price-chemotherapy-why-cancer-drugs-cost-223821525.html.

Yong, Pierre L., R. S. Saunders, and LeighAnne Olsen, eds. *The Healthcare Imperative: Lowering Costs and Improving Outcomes*. Washington, D.C.: National Academy Press, 2010. Available online at http://www.ncbi.nlm.nih.gov/books/NBK53921/.

———, eds. "Transparency of Cost and Performance," in *The Healthcare Imperative: Lowering Costs and Improving Outcomes: Workshop Series Summary*. Washington, D.C.: National Academy Press, 2010. Available online at http://www.ncbi.nlm.nih.gov/books/NBK53921/.

"Your Safer-Surgery Survival Guide: Our Ratings of 2,463 U.S. Hospitals Can Help You Find the Right One." *Consumer Reports*, July 2013. http://www.consumerreports.org/cro/magazine/2013/09/safe-surgery-survival-guide/index.htm.

Zietman, Anthony L. "Falsification, Fabrication, and Plagiarism: The Unholy Trinity of Scientific Writing." *International Journal of Radiation Oncology* 87, no. 2 (October 1, 2013): 225–27. http://www.elsevier.com/connect/falsification-fabrication-and-plagiarism-the-unholy-trinity-of-scientific-writing.

INDEX

ABOUT THE AUTHOR

John Leifer brings a unique perspective to the challenges facing America's health care system. It is a perspective garnered through thirty years of work across multiple sectors of the health care industry—from health systems to health insurers, from health information technology to governmental organizations. Most recently, Leifer served as senior vice president for a ten-hospital system in the Midwest. In the early 1990s Leifer founded and published *The Leifer Report*, a health care publication that featured contributors ranging from President Bill Clinton to Newt Gingrich. He has written extensively on health care issues and has been published in newspapers and magazines such as *Modern Healthcare, Hospitals & Health Networks, Washington Monthly*, and the *Kansas City Star*. Leifer has also been profiled throughout the years in several prominent magazines, including *Money* and *Fortune*. Leifer also served as the first executive in residence for the University of Kansas School of Medicine's Health Policy and Management Program, where he was the recipient of the Kansas Health Foundation Excellence in Teaching Award. Mr. Leifer may be contacted at jleifer@leifer.com.